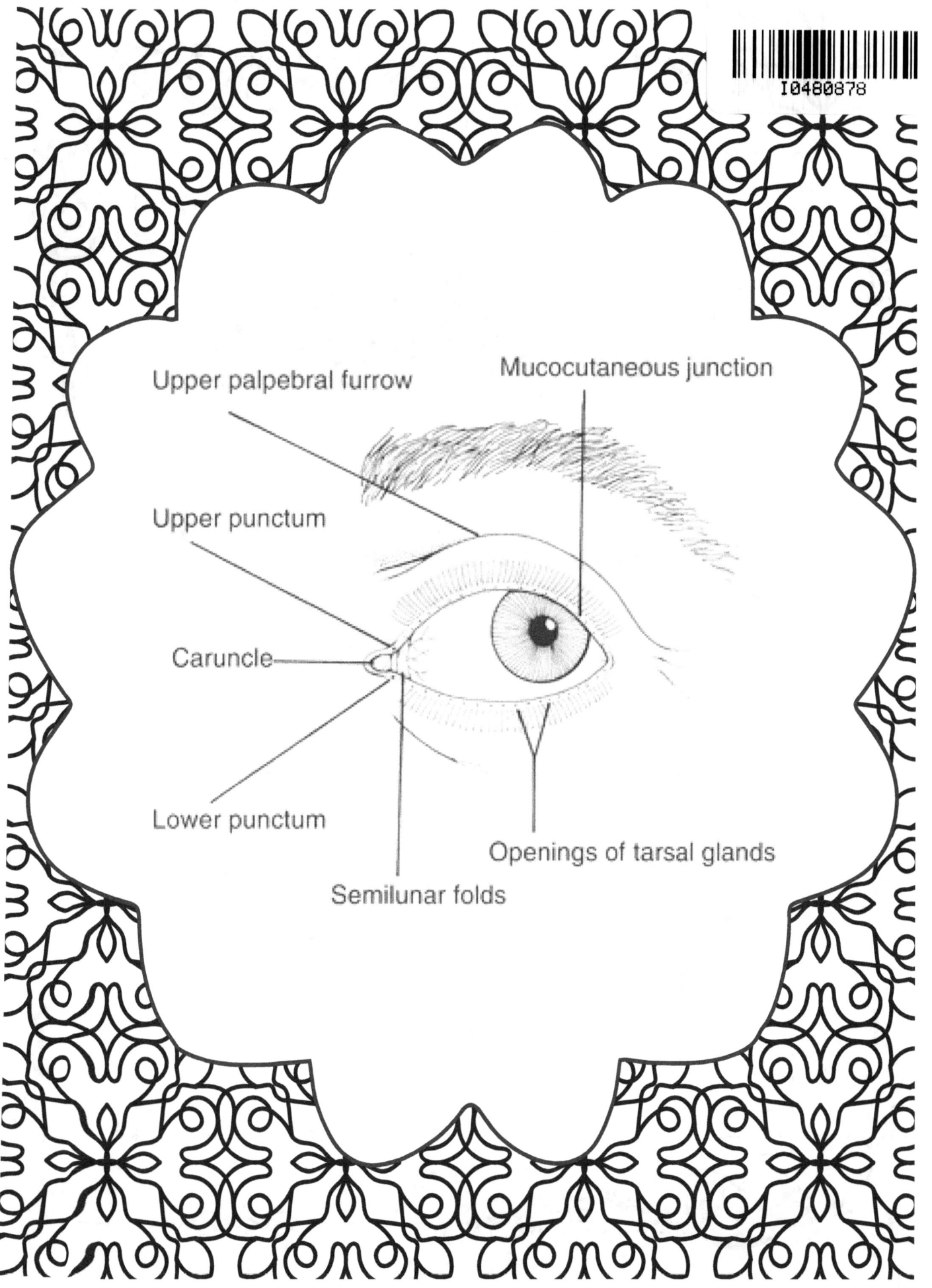

Upper palpebral furrow

Mucocutaneous junction

Upper punctum

Caruncle

Lower punctum

Openings of tarsal glands

Semilunar folds

This Book Belongs To

_____

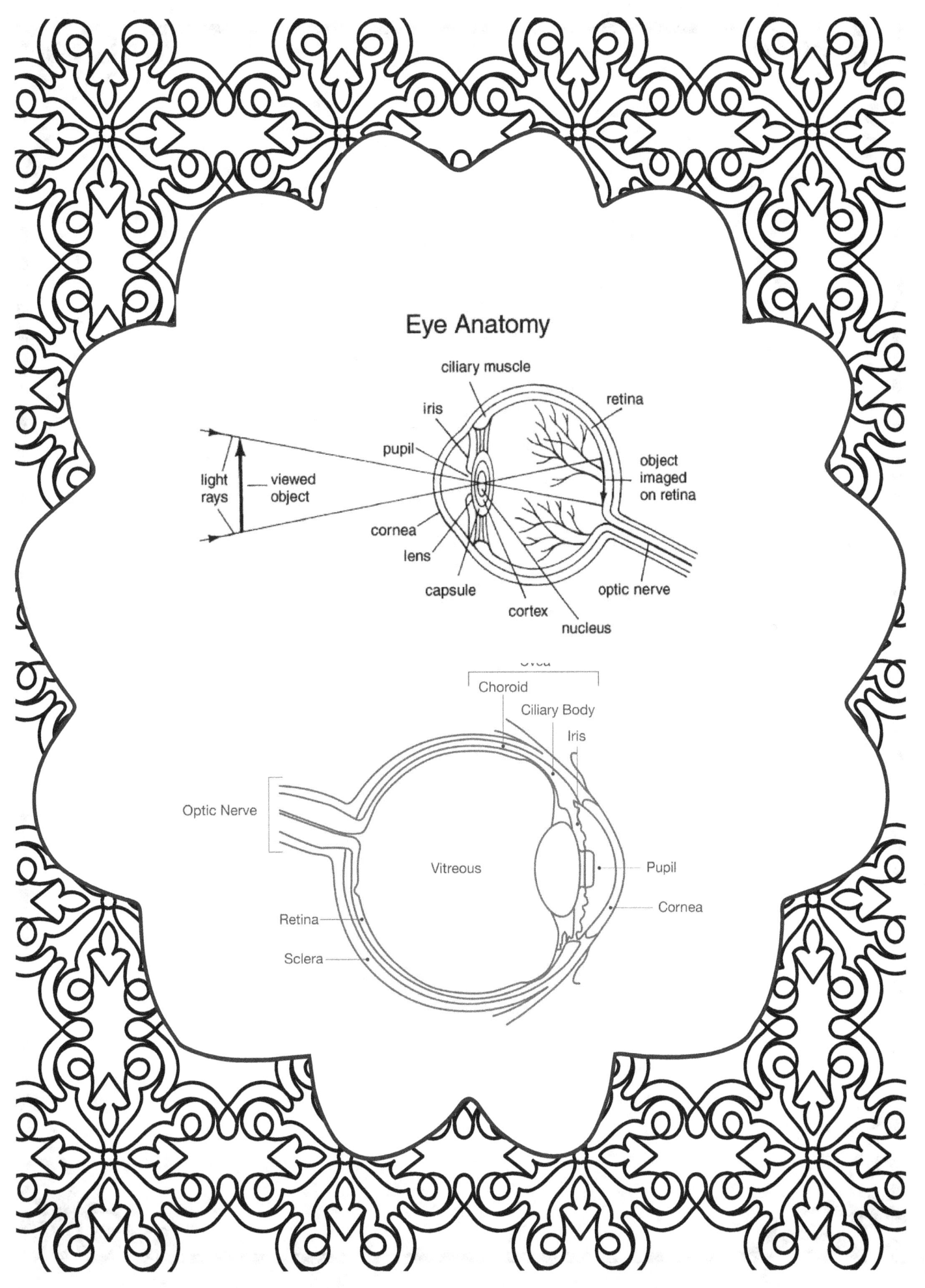

Eye Anatomy

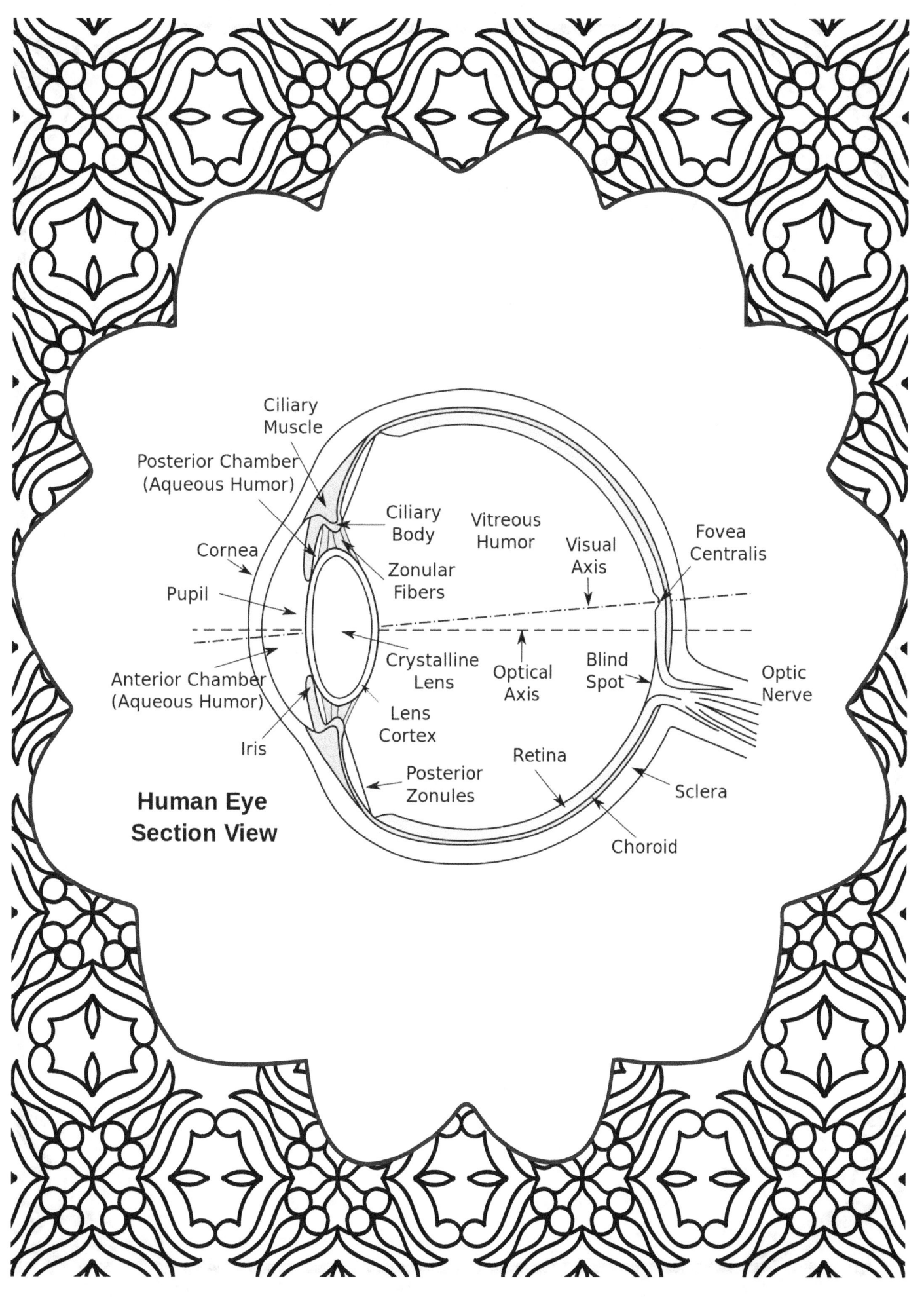

Human Eye
Section View

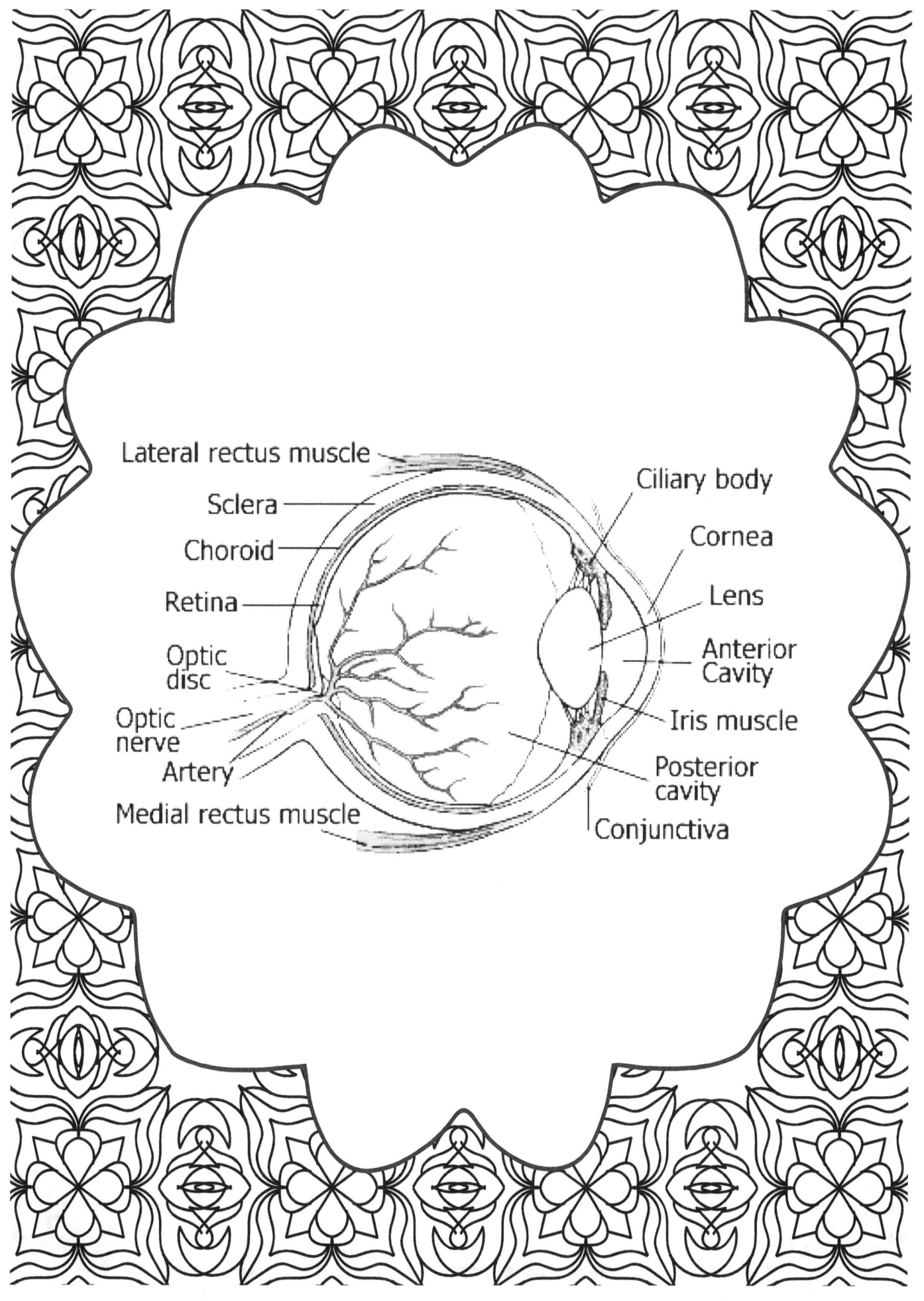

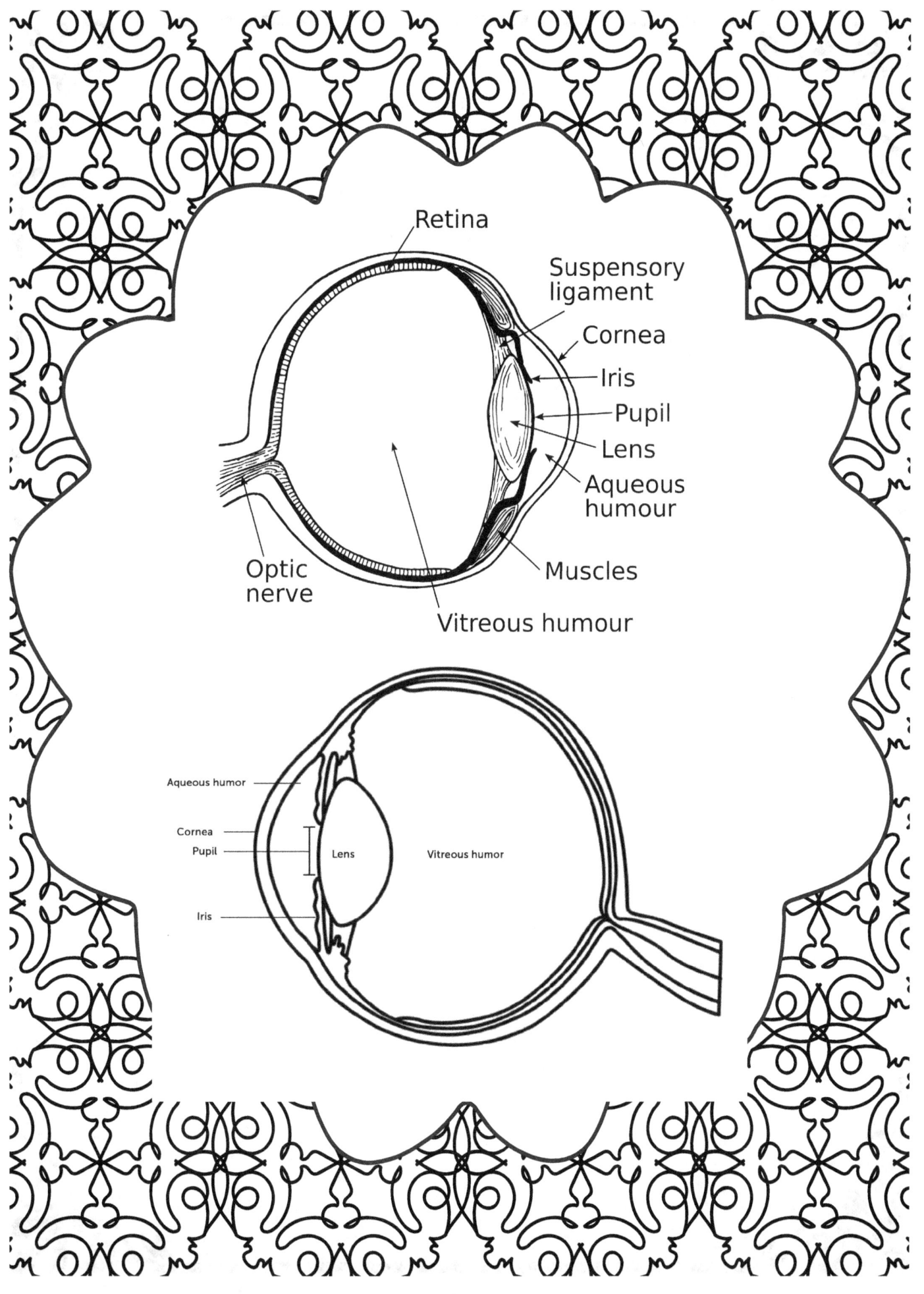

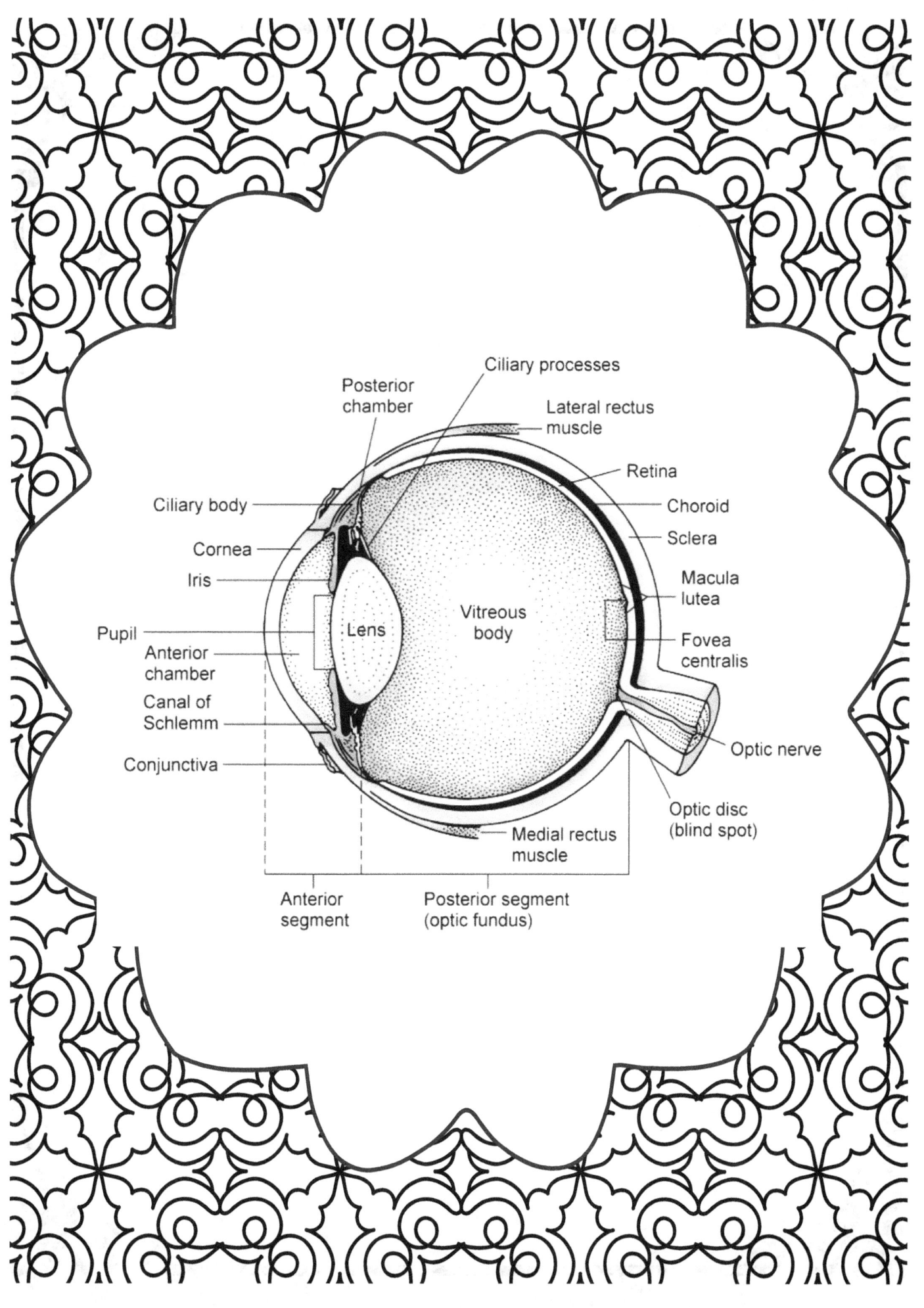

Anatomy of the Human Eye

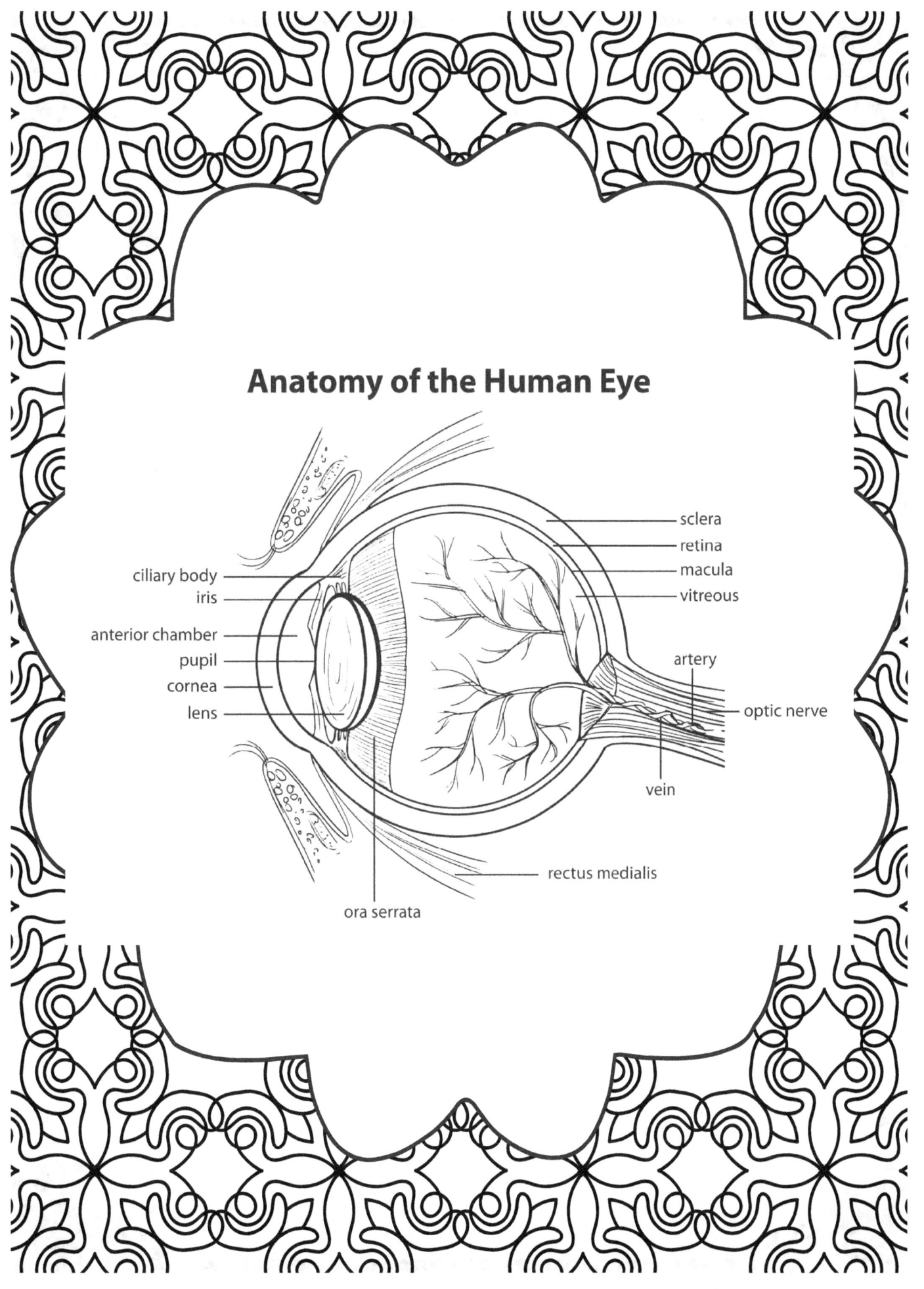

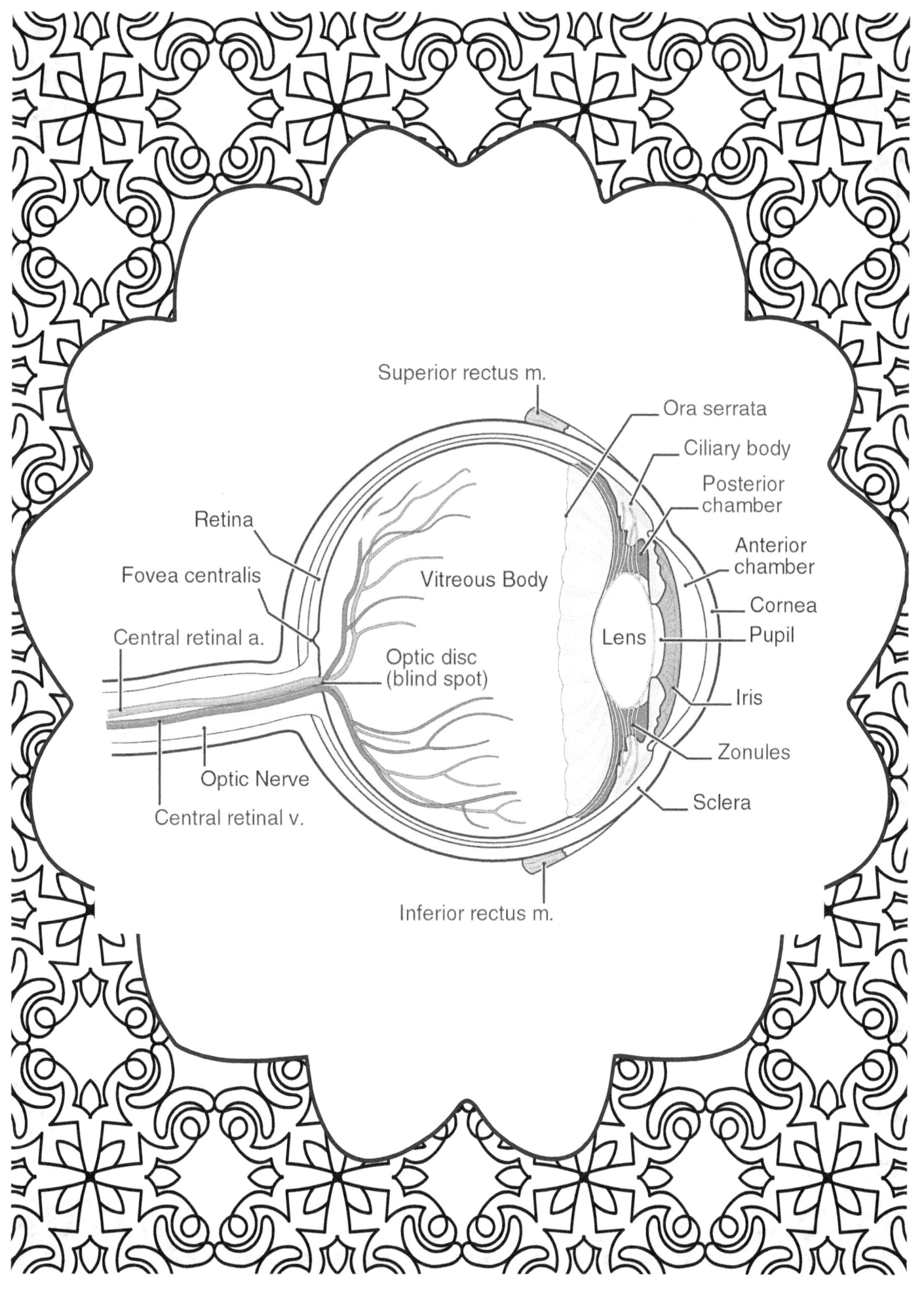

Superior rectus m.

Ora serrata

Ciliary body

Posterior chamber

Anterior chamber

Cornea

Pupil

Iris

Zonules

Sclera

Lens

Vitreous Body

Retina

Fovea centralis

Central retinal a.

Optic disc (blind spot)

Optic Nerve

Central retinal v.

Inferior rectus m.

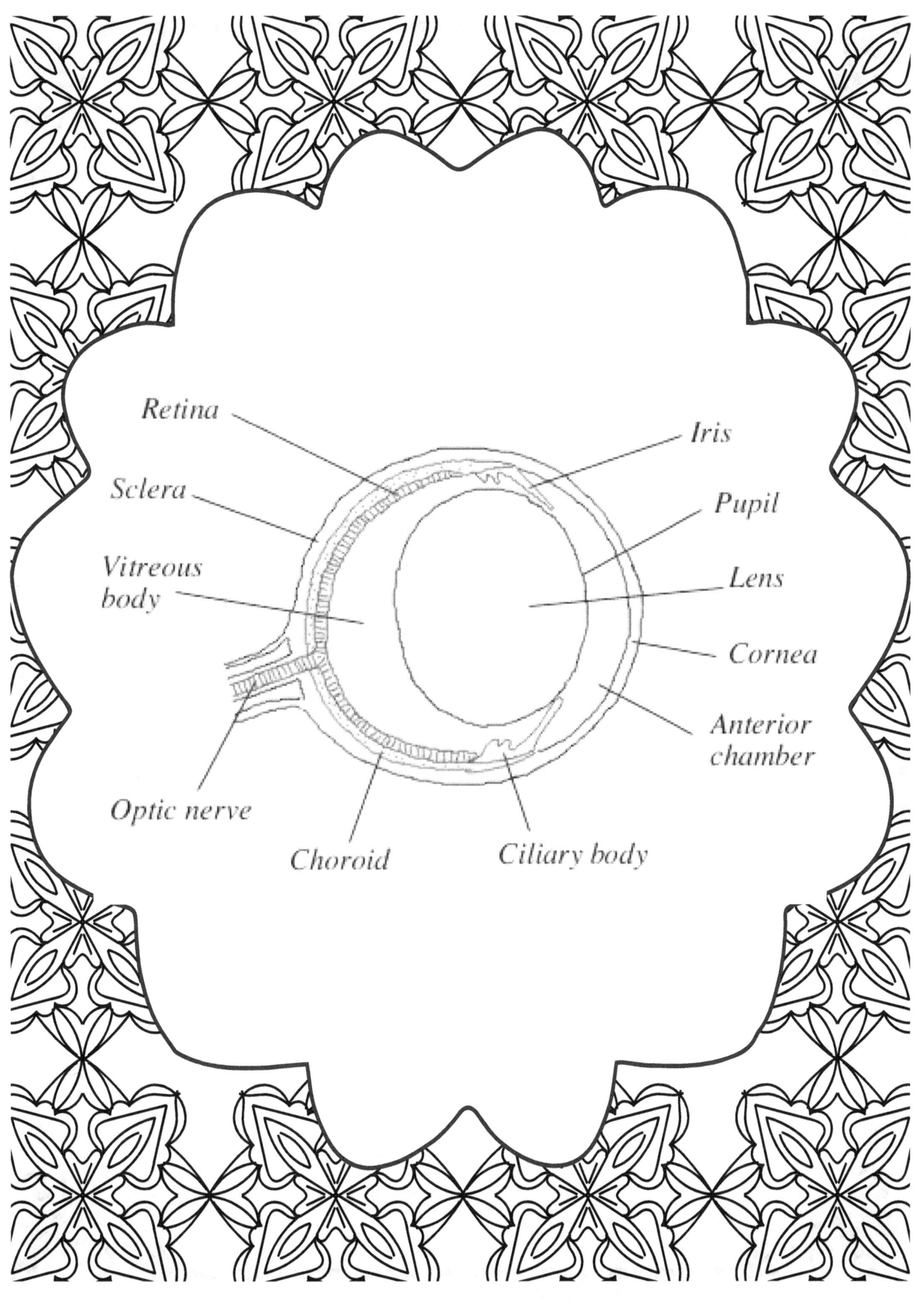

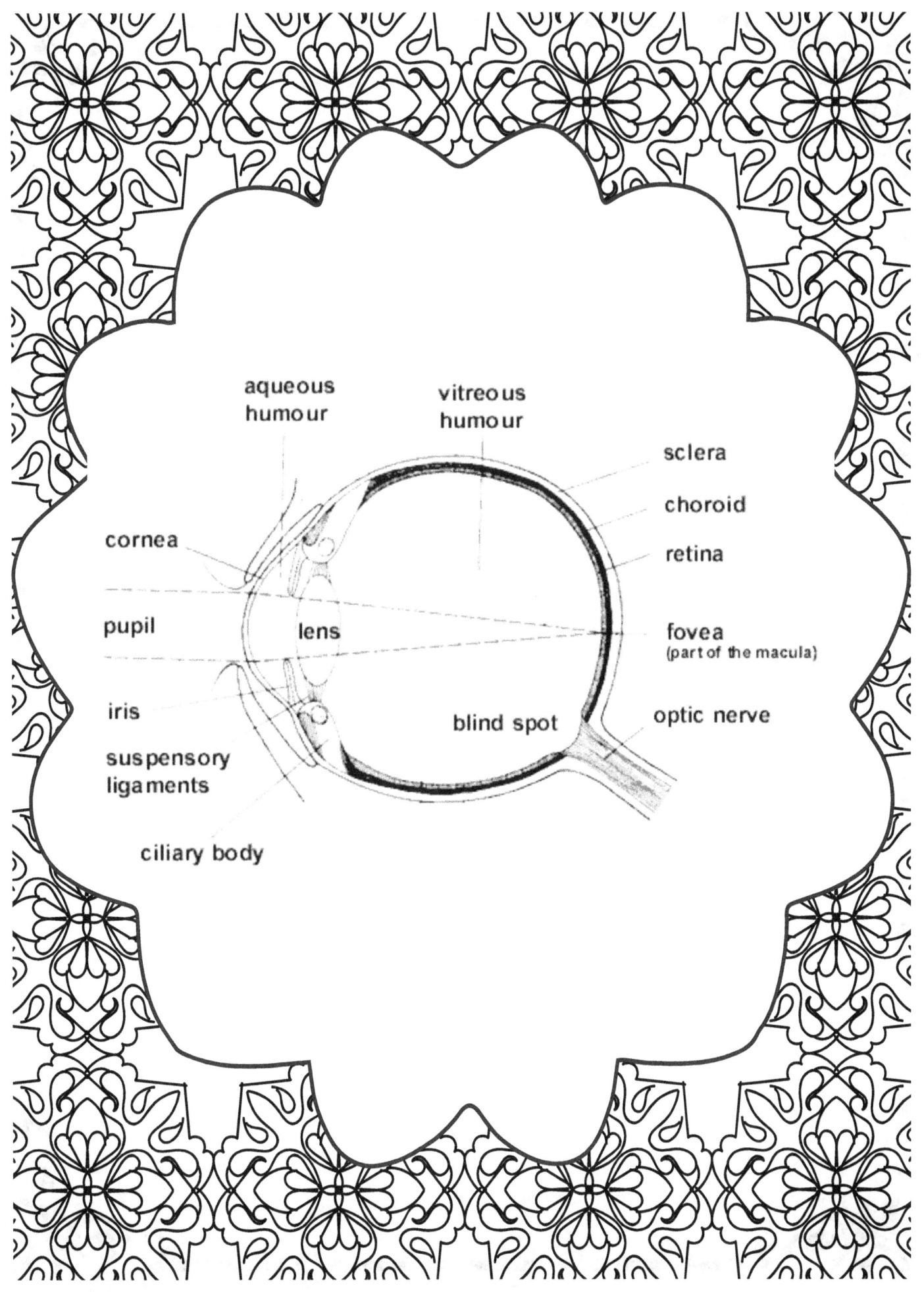

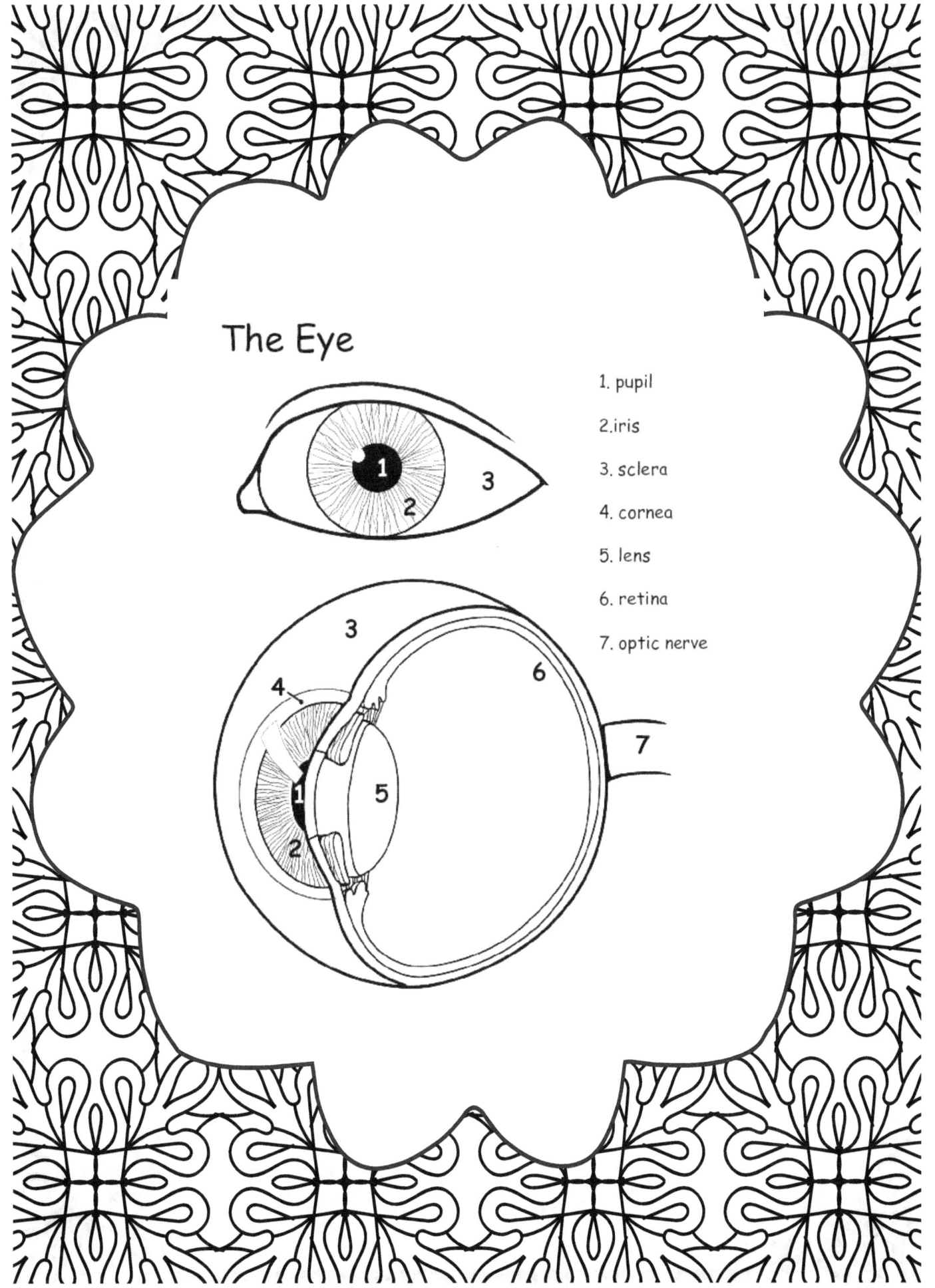

The Eye

1. pupil

2. iris

3. sclera

4. cornea

5. lens

6. retina

7. optic nerve

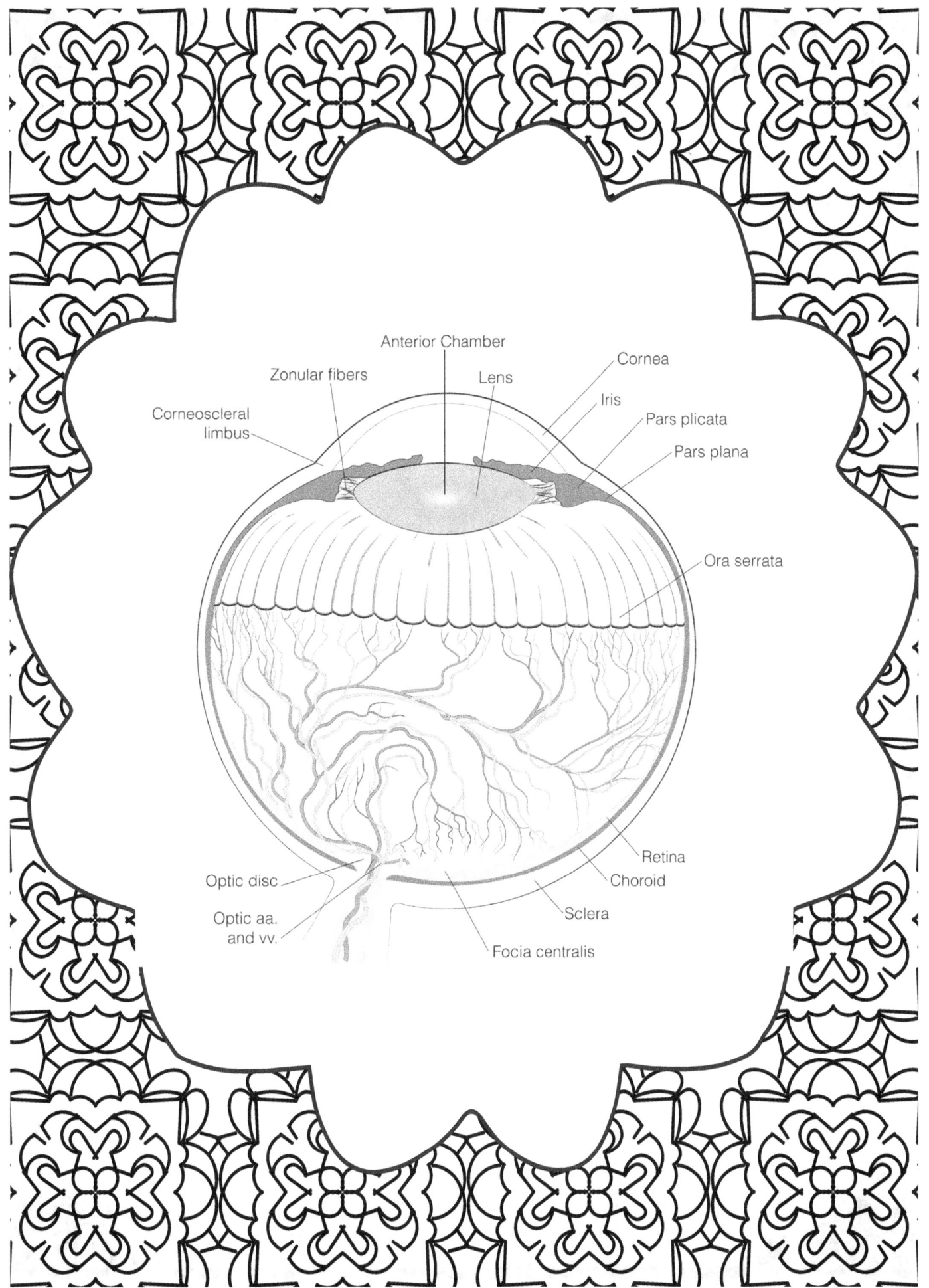

Anterior Chamber

Zonular fibers

Cornea

Iris

Corneoscleral
limbus

Lens

Pars plicata

Pars plana

Ora serrata

Retina

Choroid

Optic disc

Sclera

Optic aa.
and vv.

Focia centralis

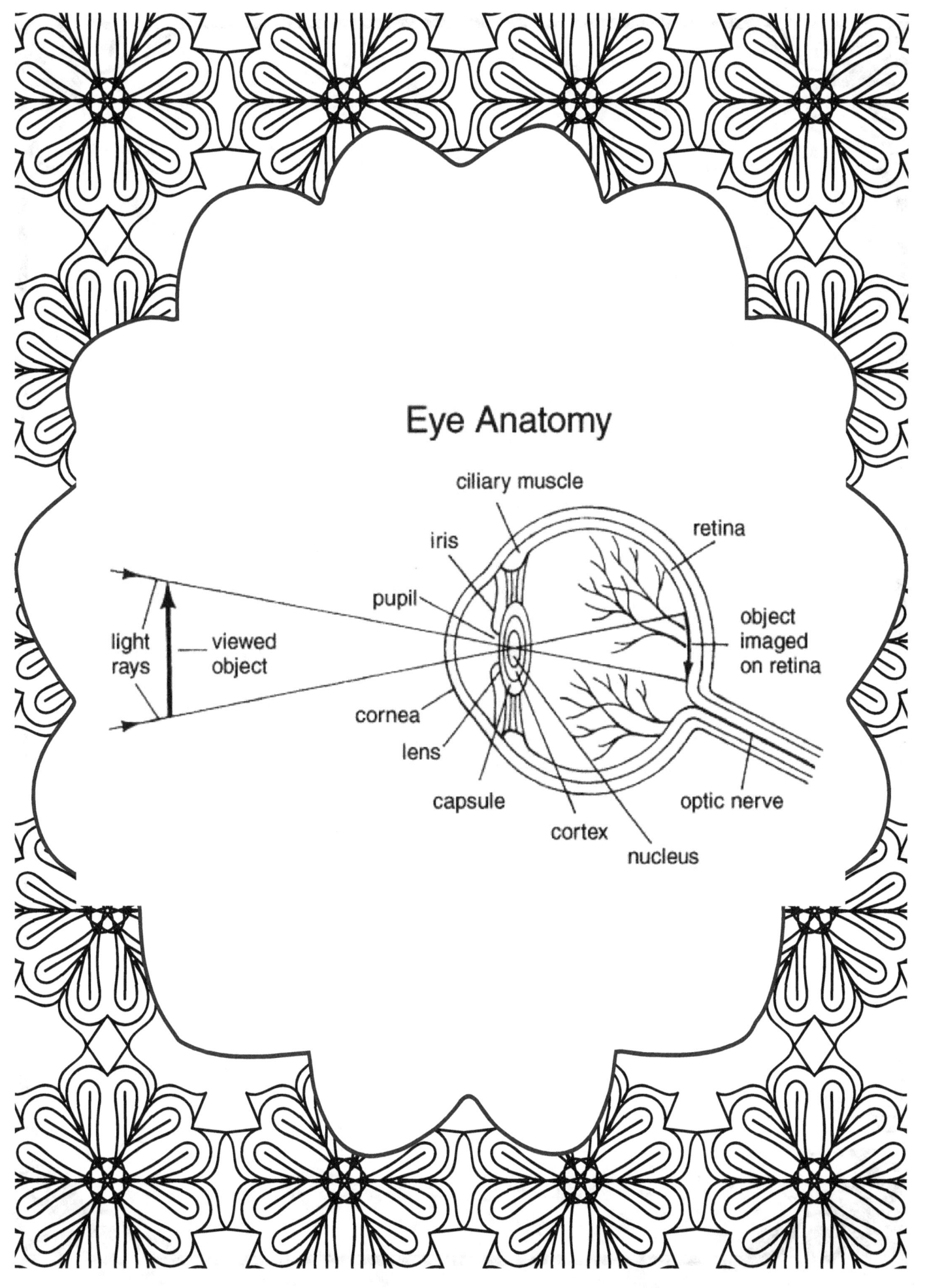

Eye Anatomy

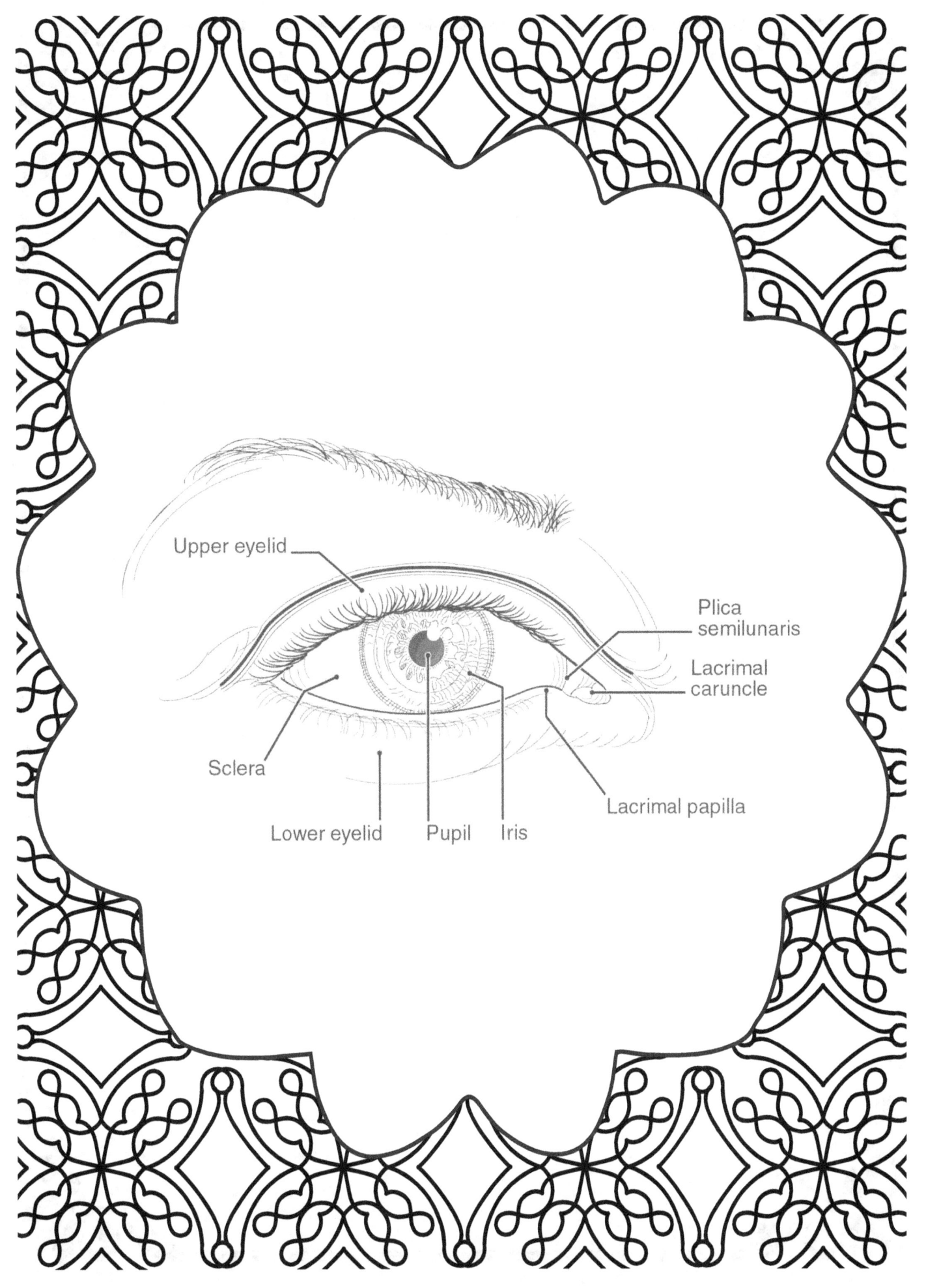

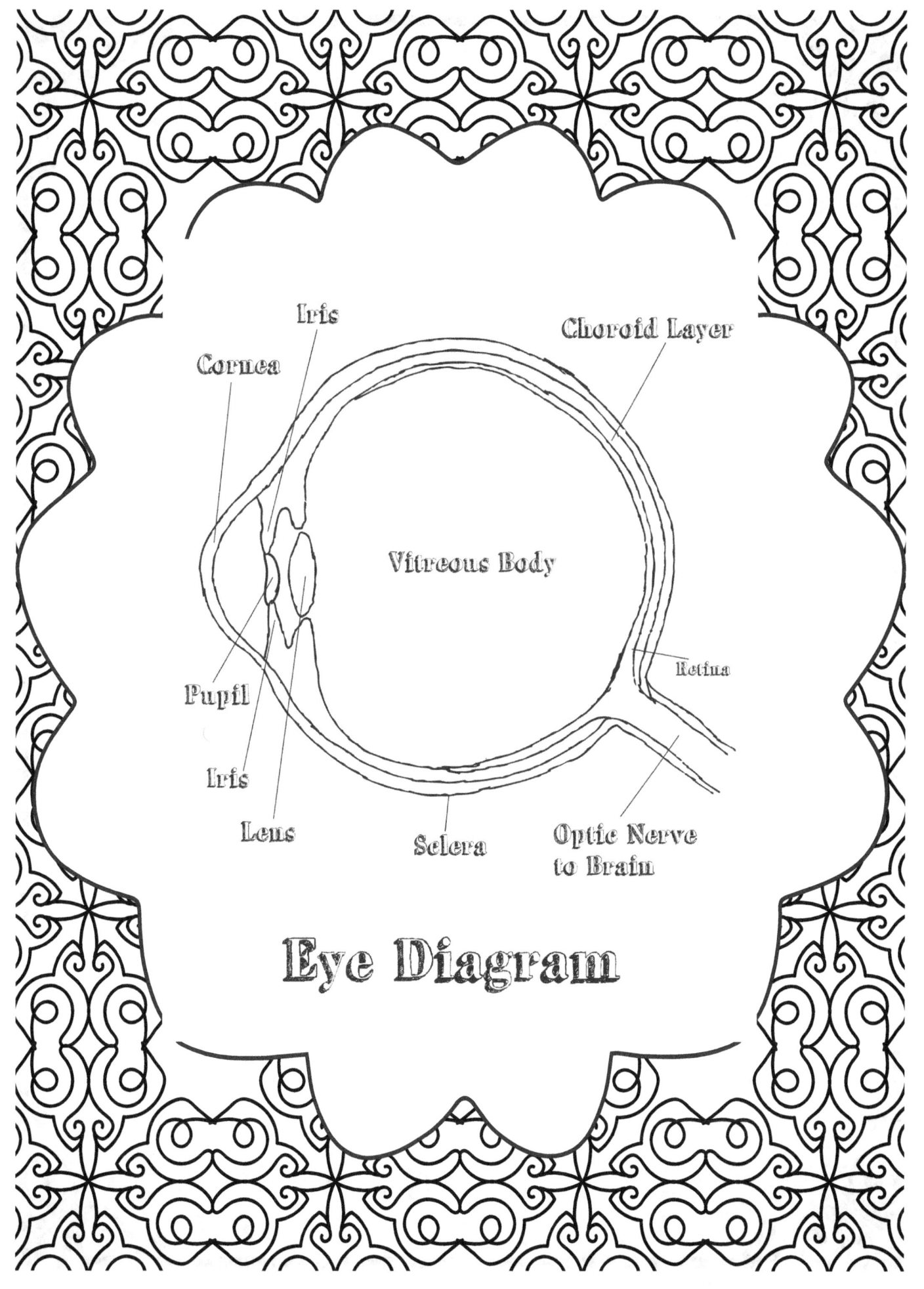

Iris

Cornea

Choroid Layer

Vitreous Body

Retina

Pupil

Iris

Optic Nerve
to Brain

Lens

Sclera

Eye Diagram

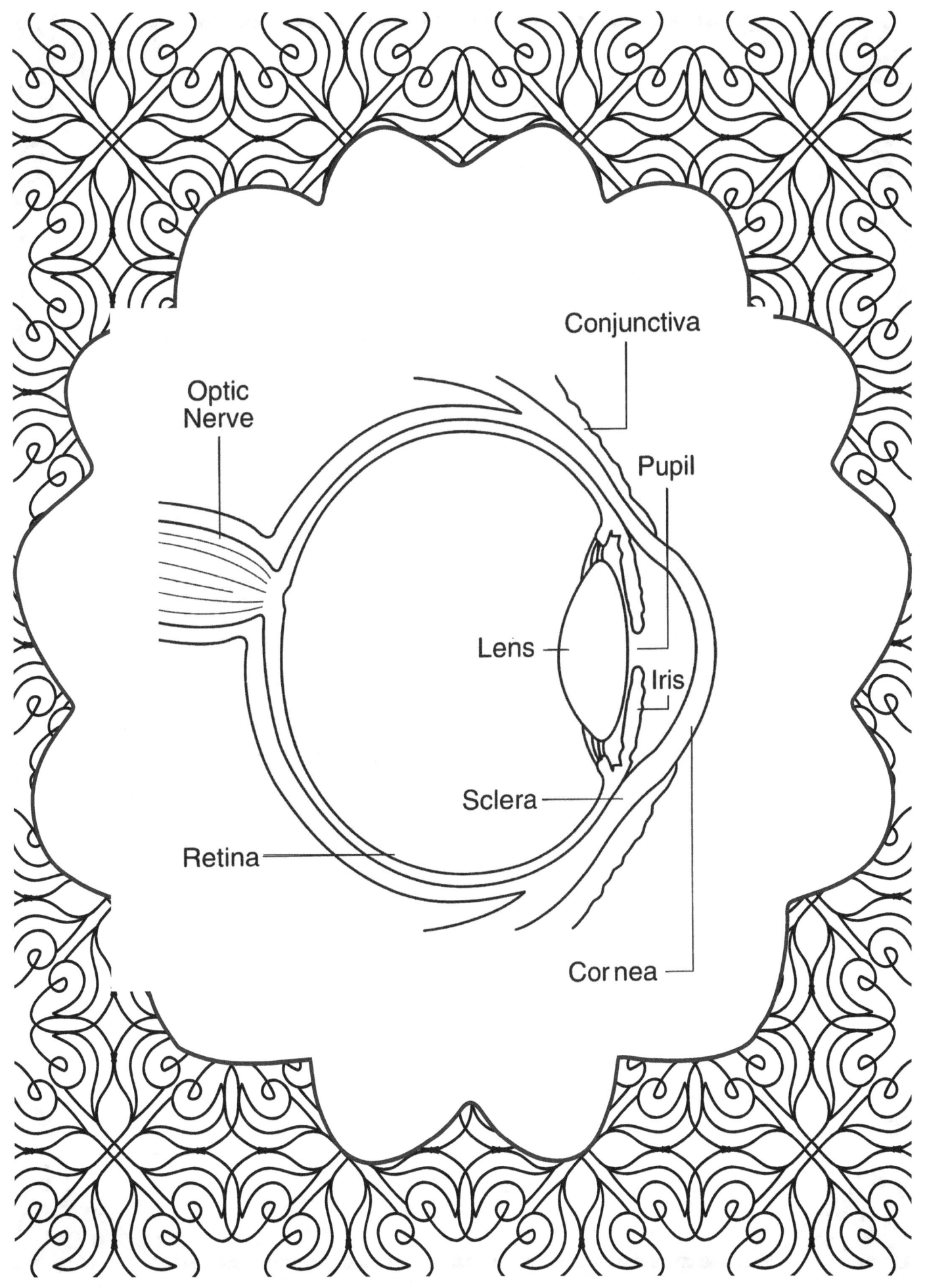

Optic
Nerve

Conjunctiva

Pupil

Lens

Iris

Sclera

Retina

Cornea

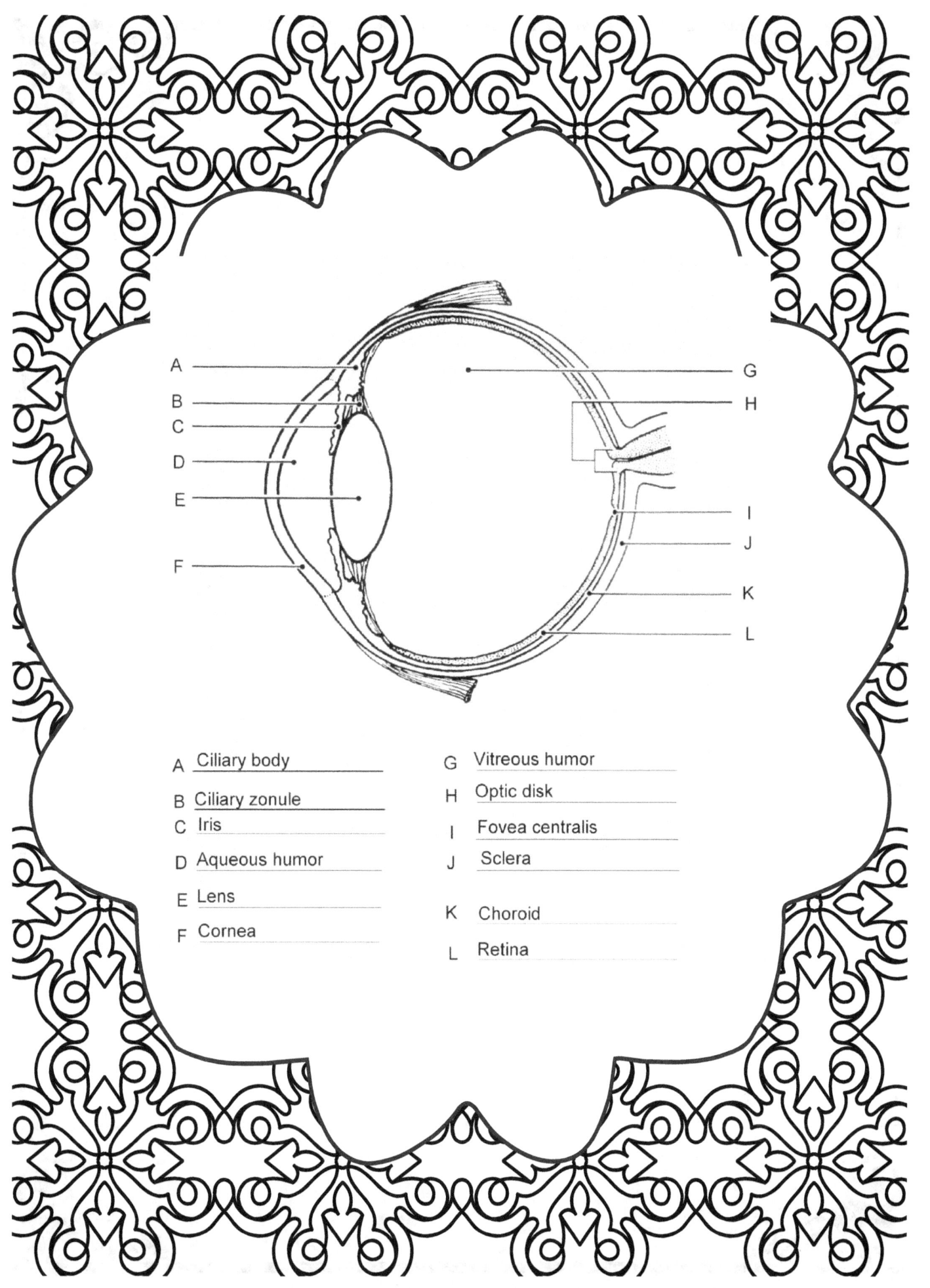

A   Ciliary body   G   Vitreous humor

B   Ciliary zonule   H   Optic disk

C   Iris   I   Fovea centralis

D   Aqueous humor   J   Sclera

E   Lens

F   Cornea   K   Choroid

                                          L   Retina

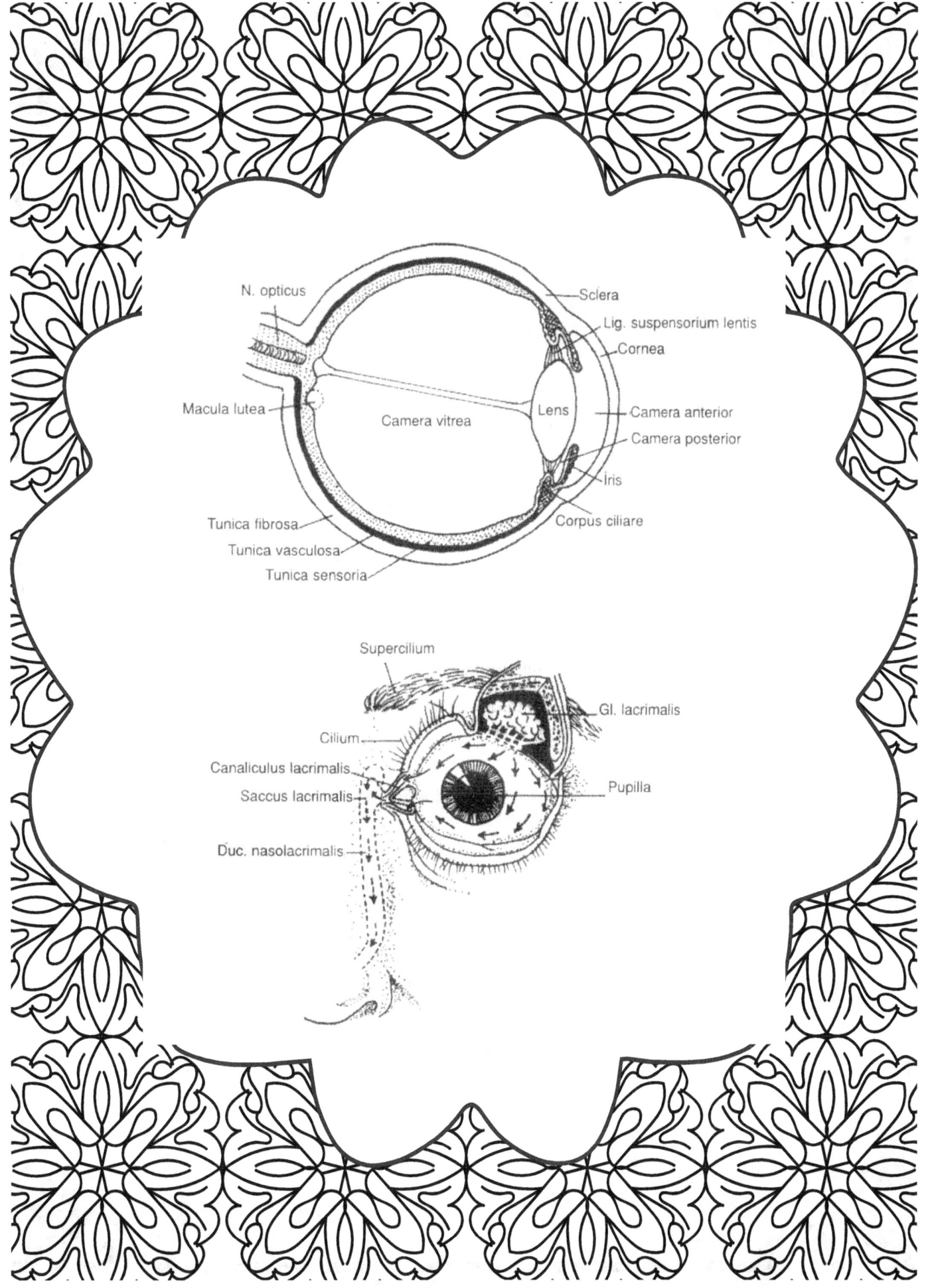

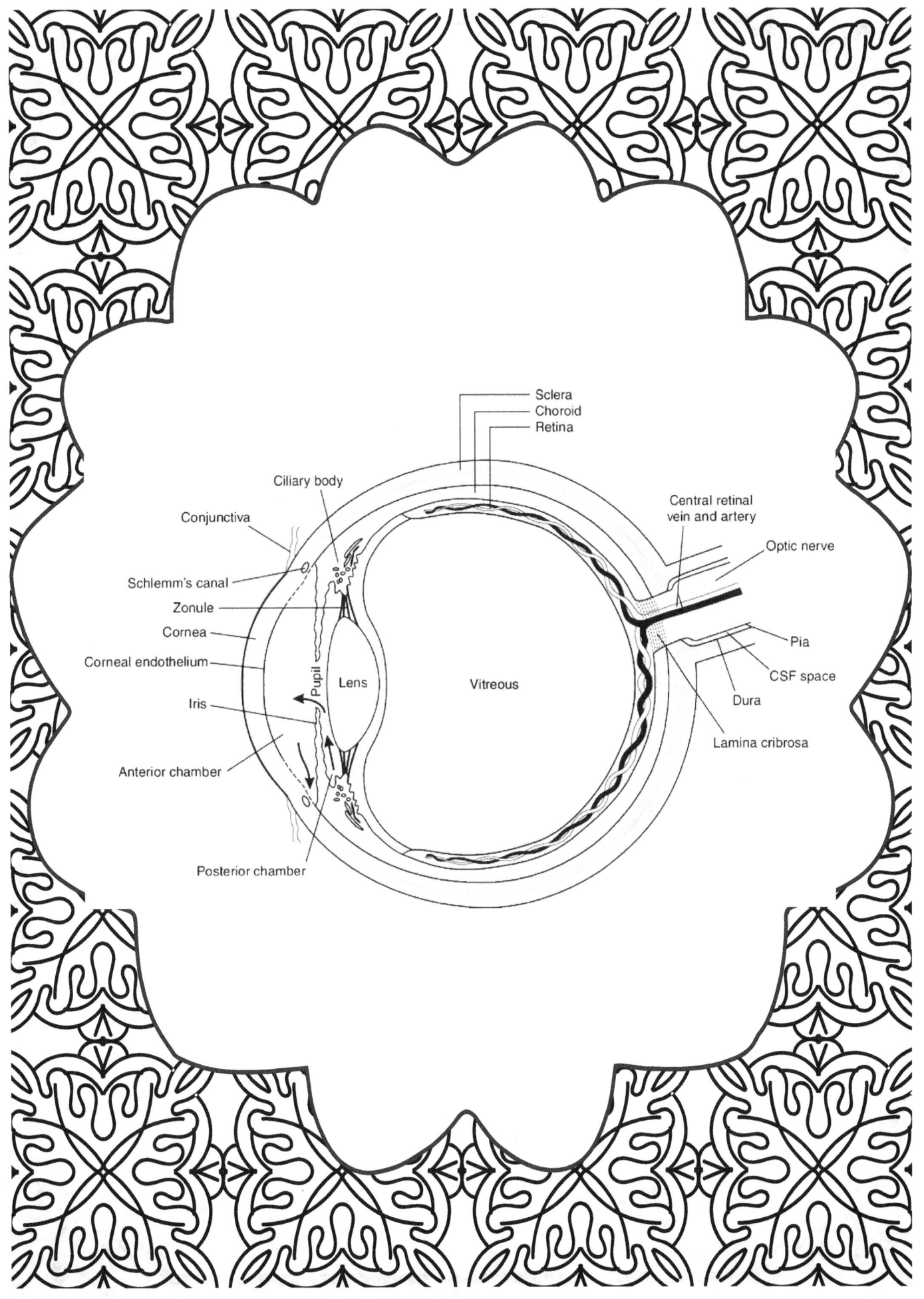

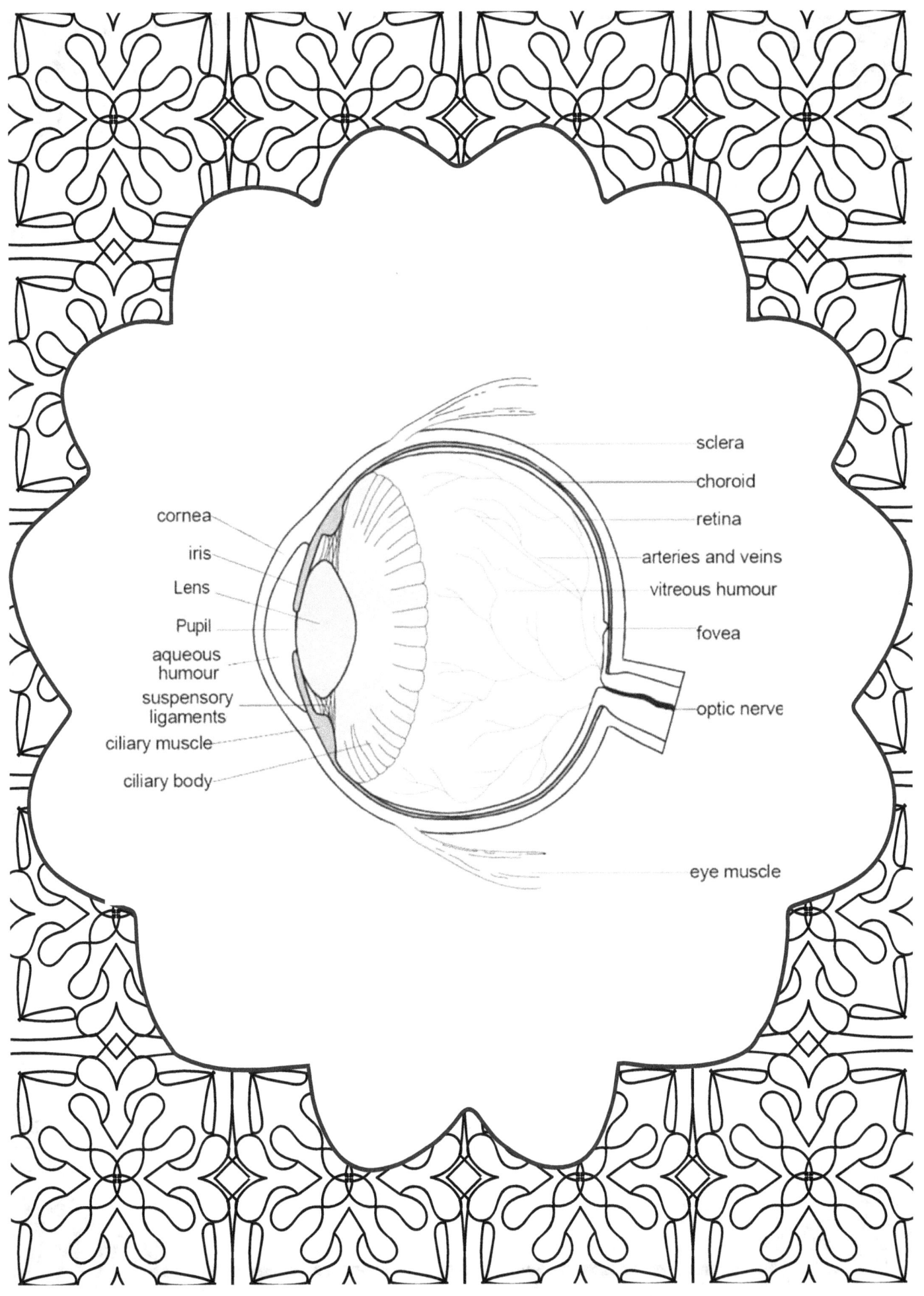

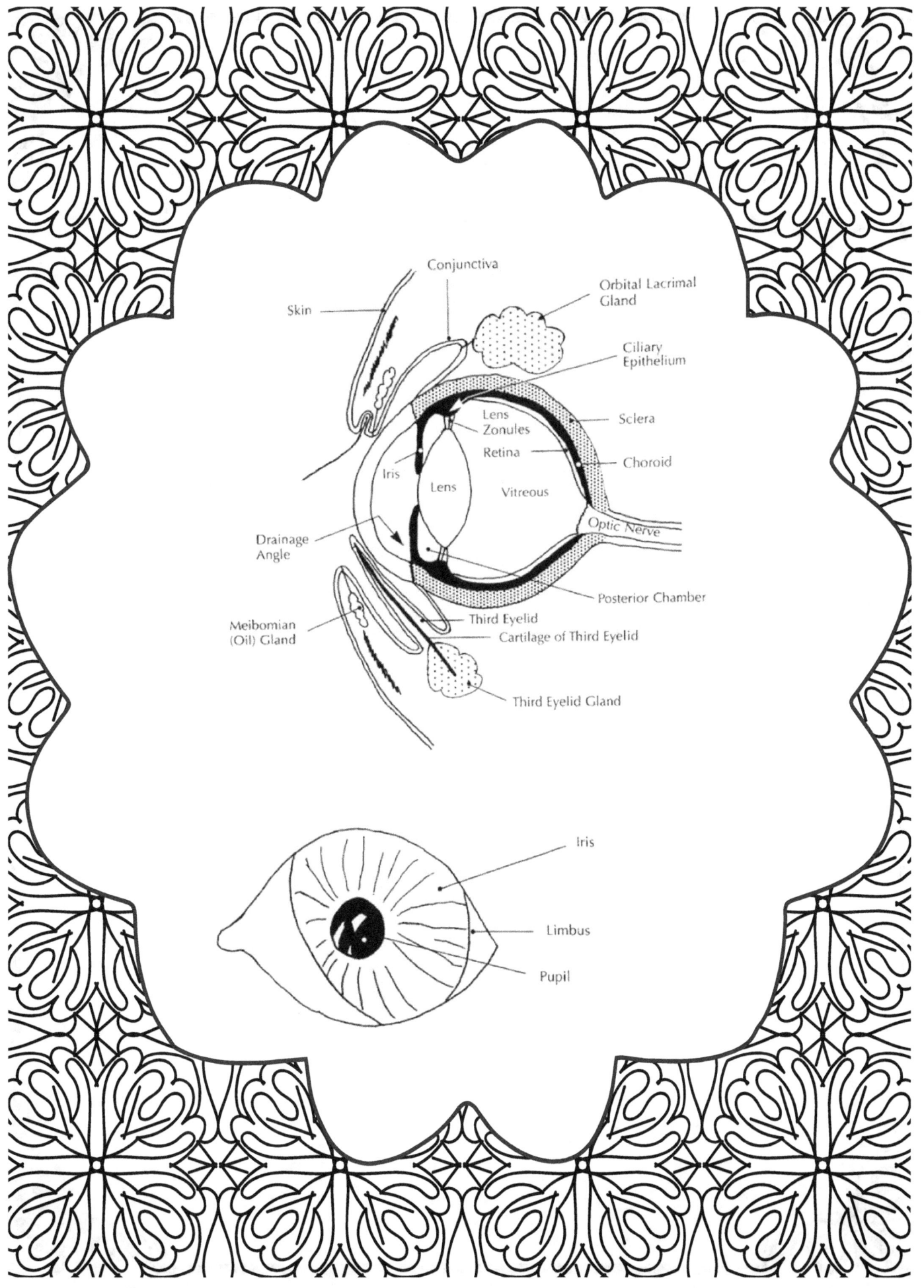

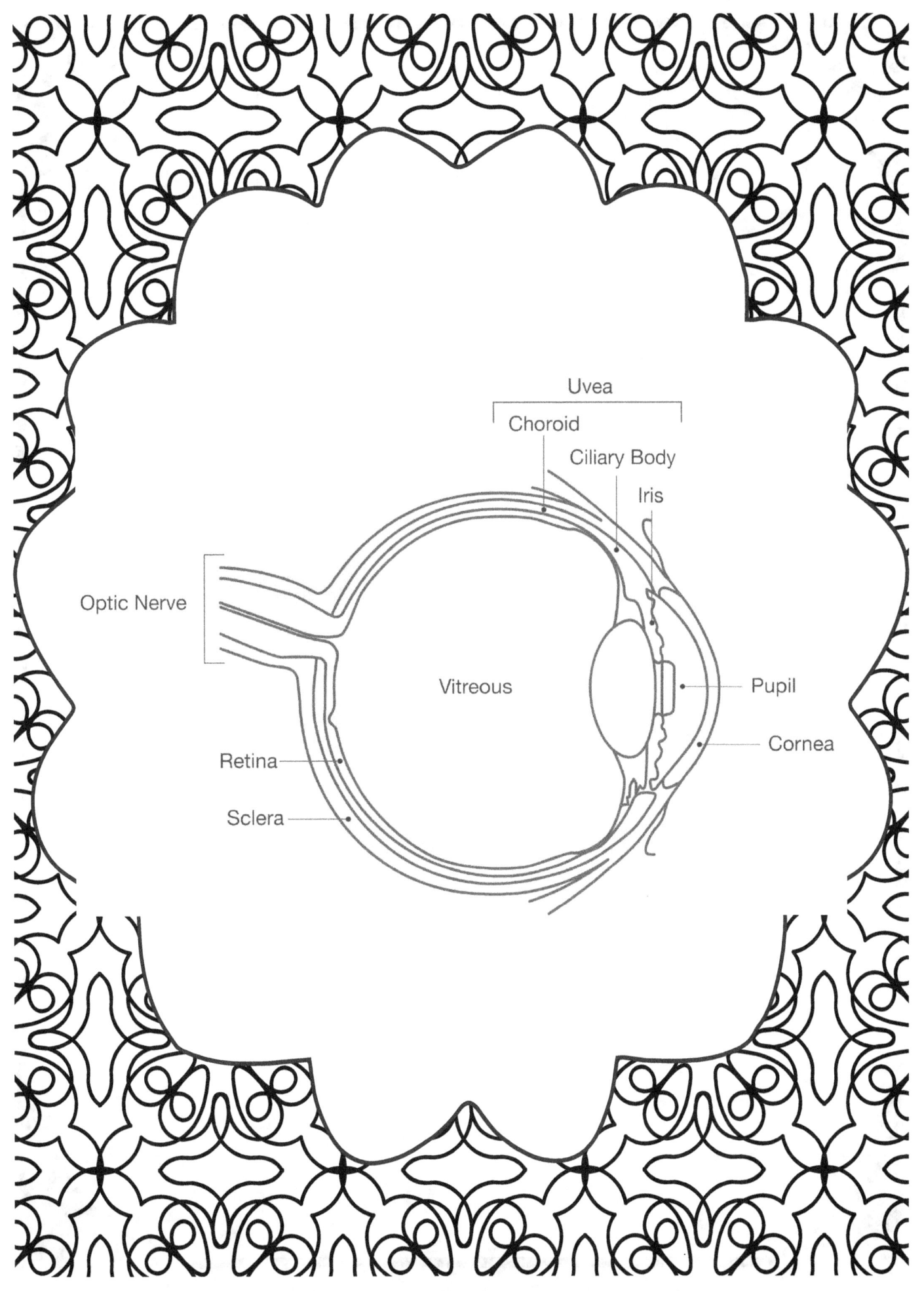

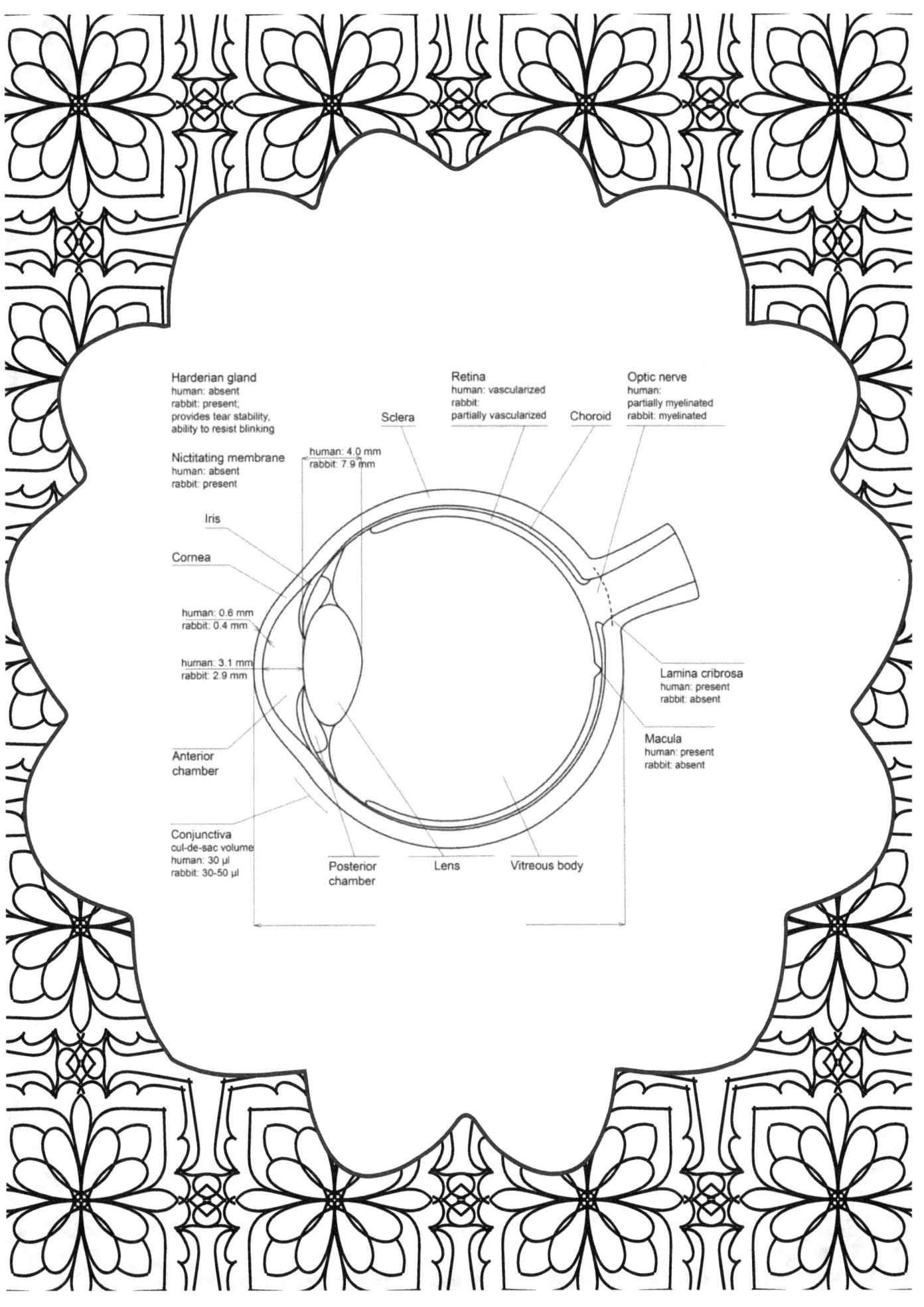

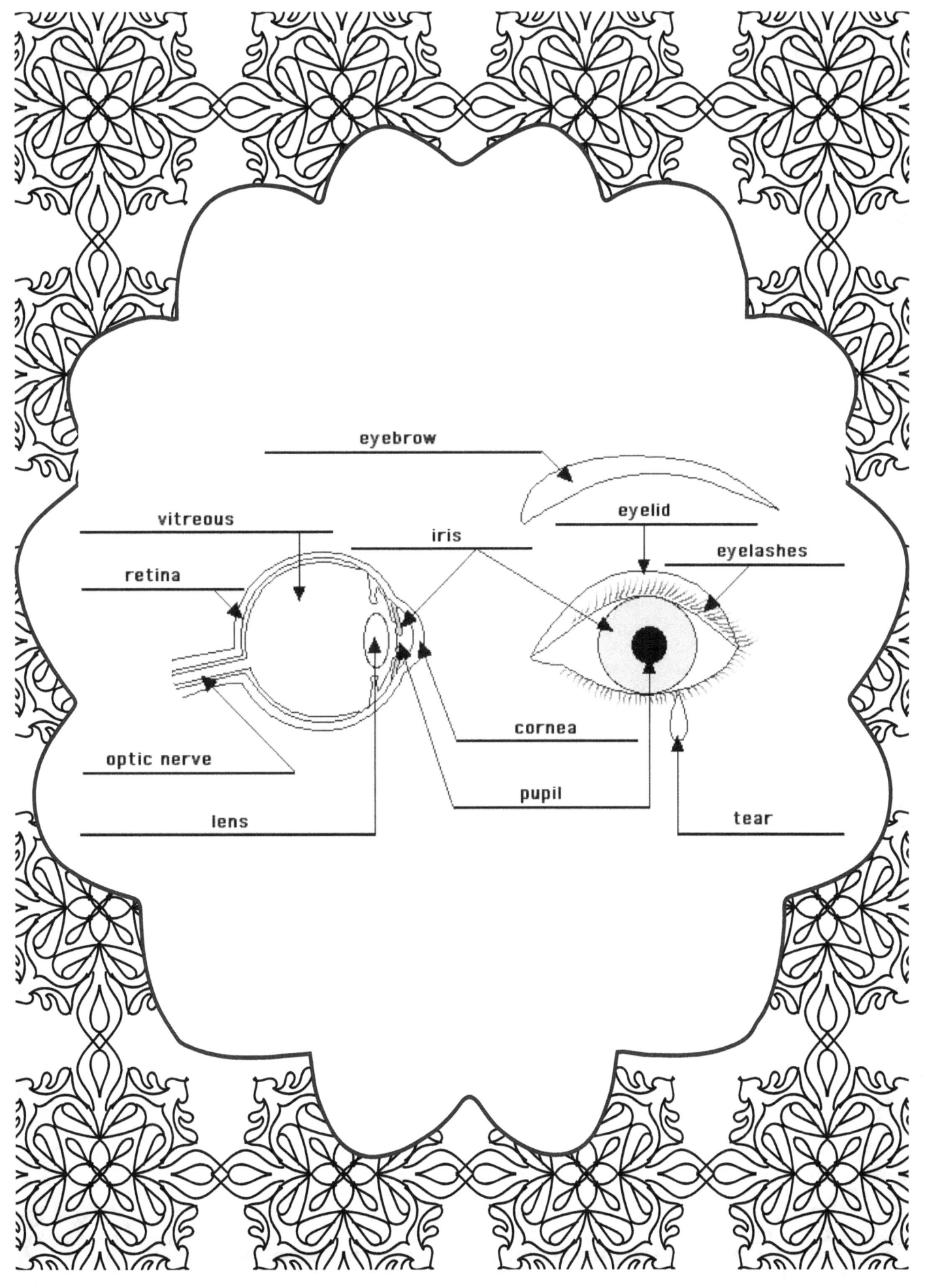

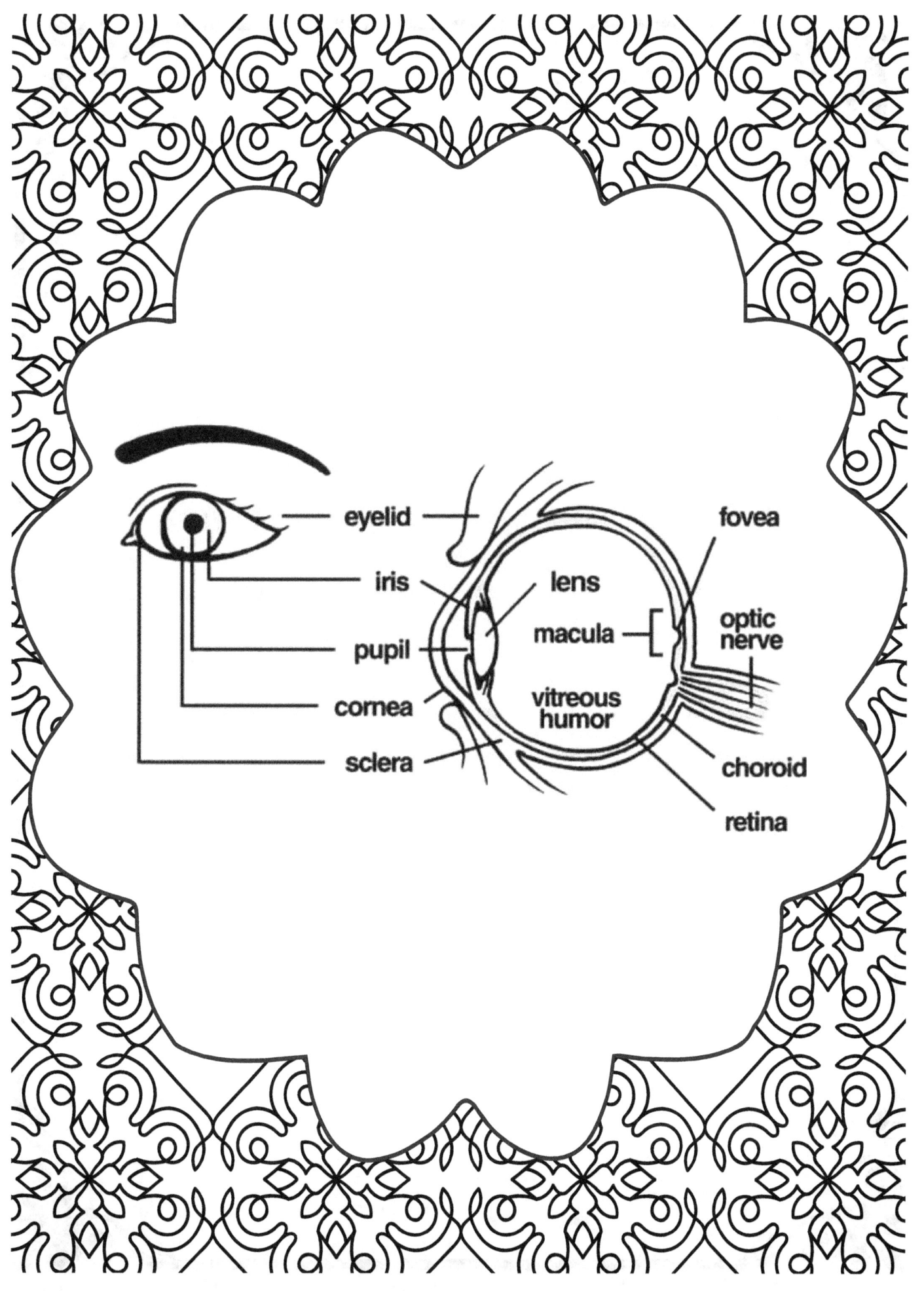

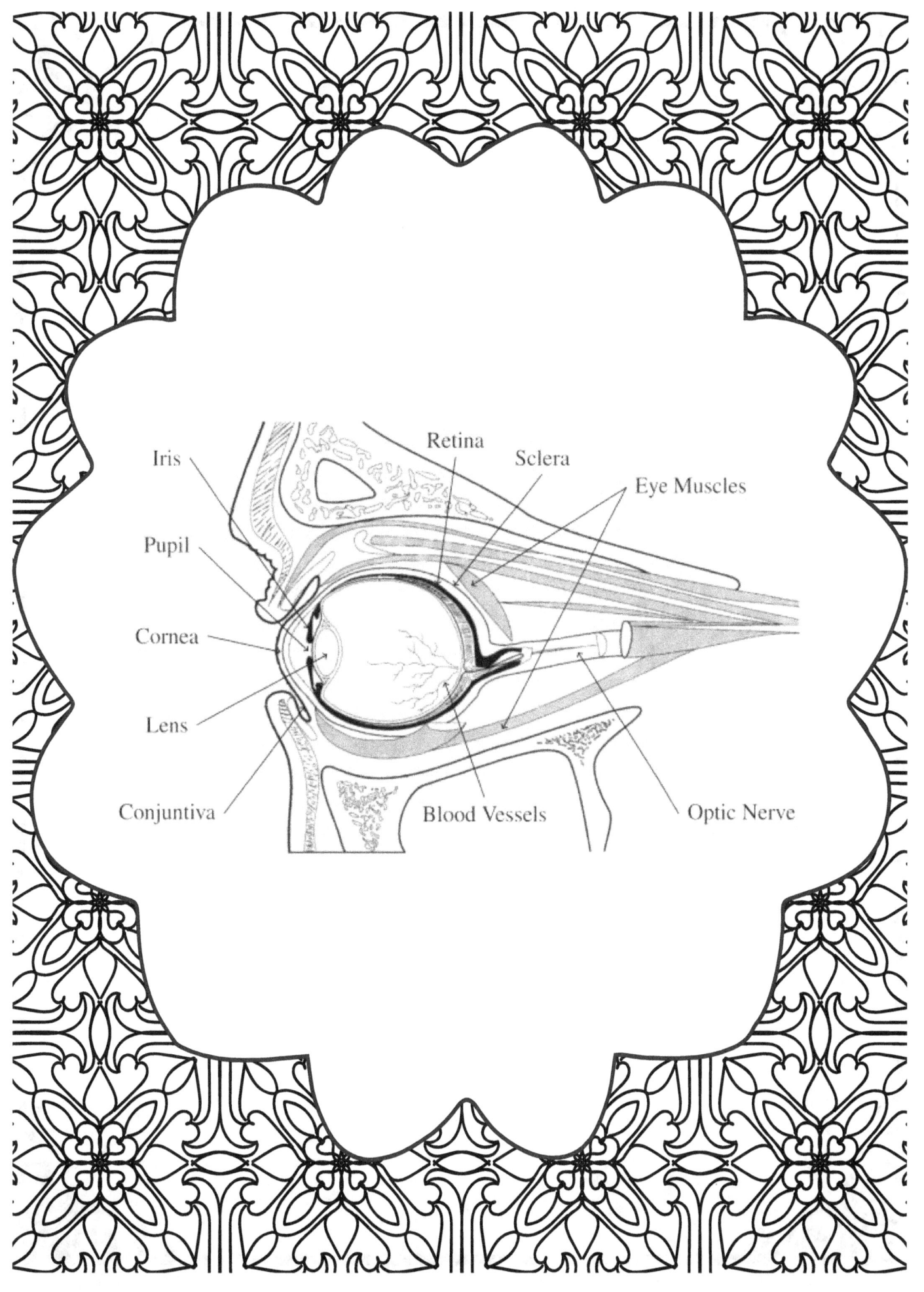

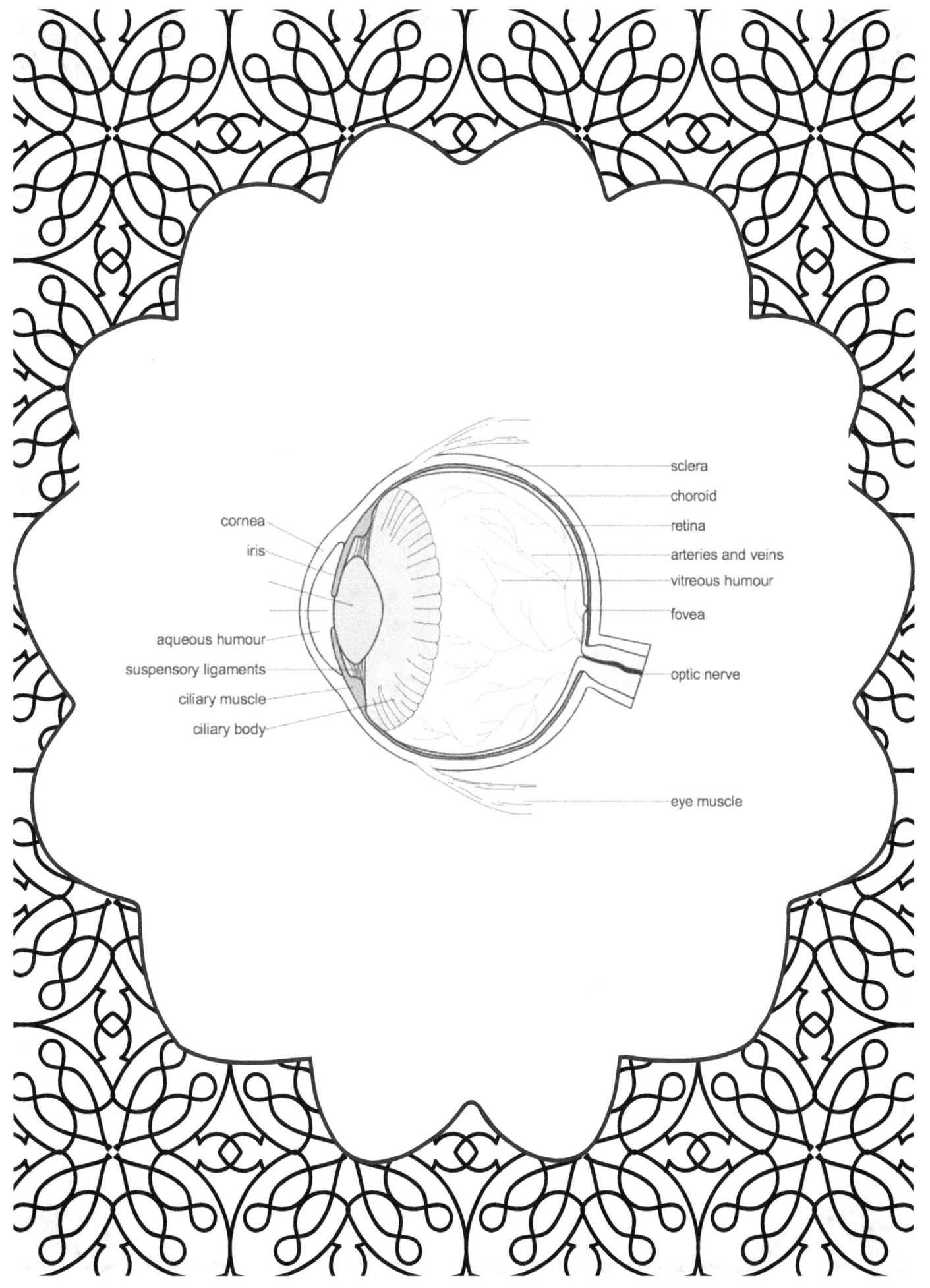

sclera

choroid

retina

arteries and veins

vitreous humour

fovea

cornea

iris

optic nerve

aqueous humour

suspensory ligaments

ciliary muscle

ciliary body

eye muscle

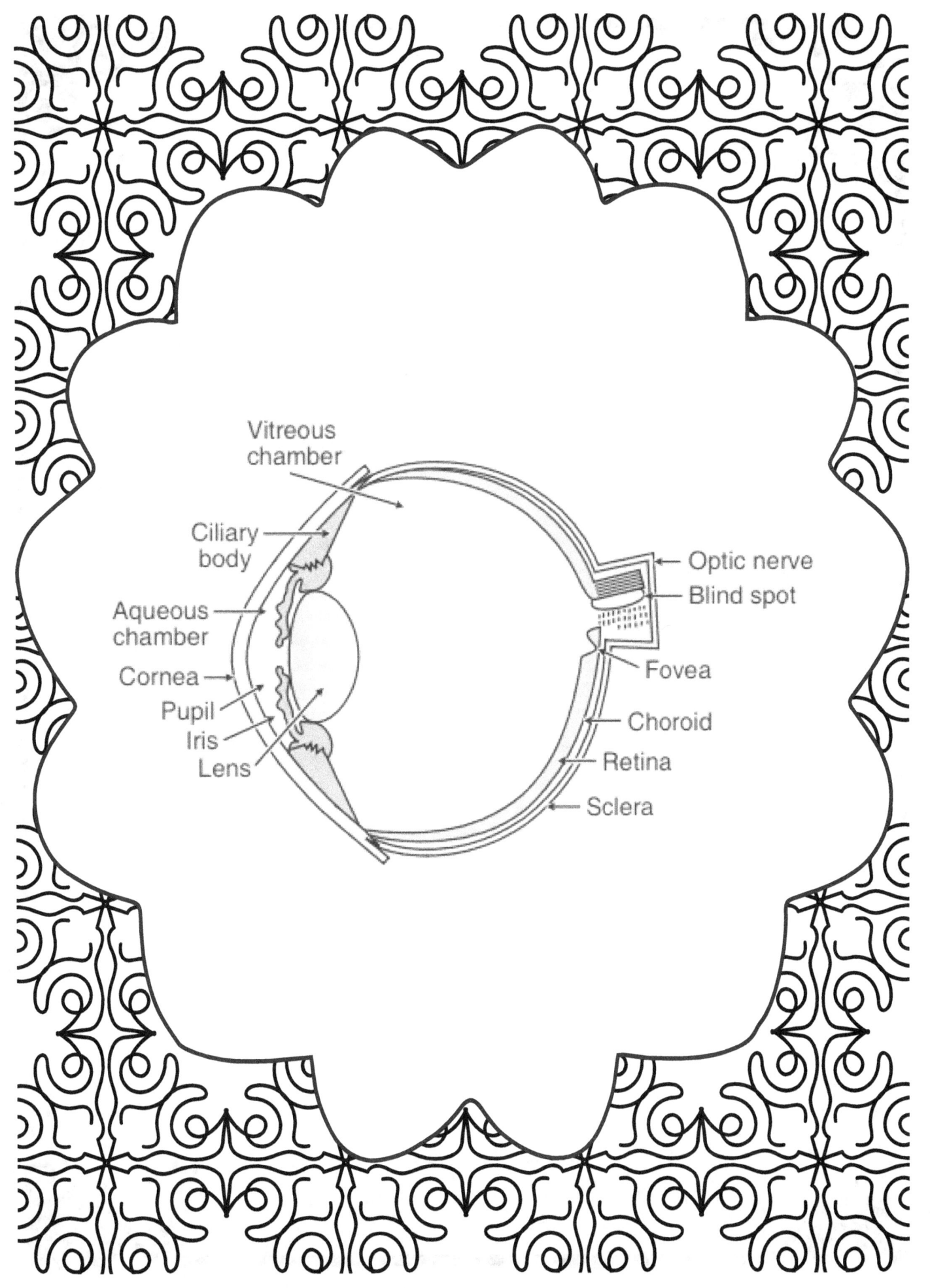

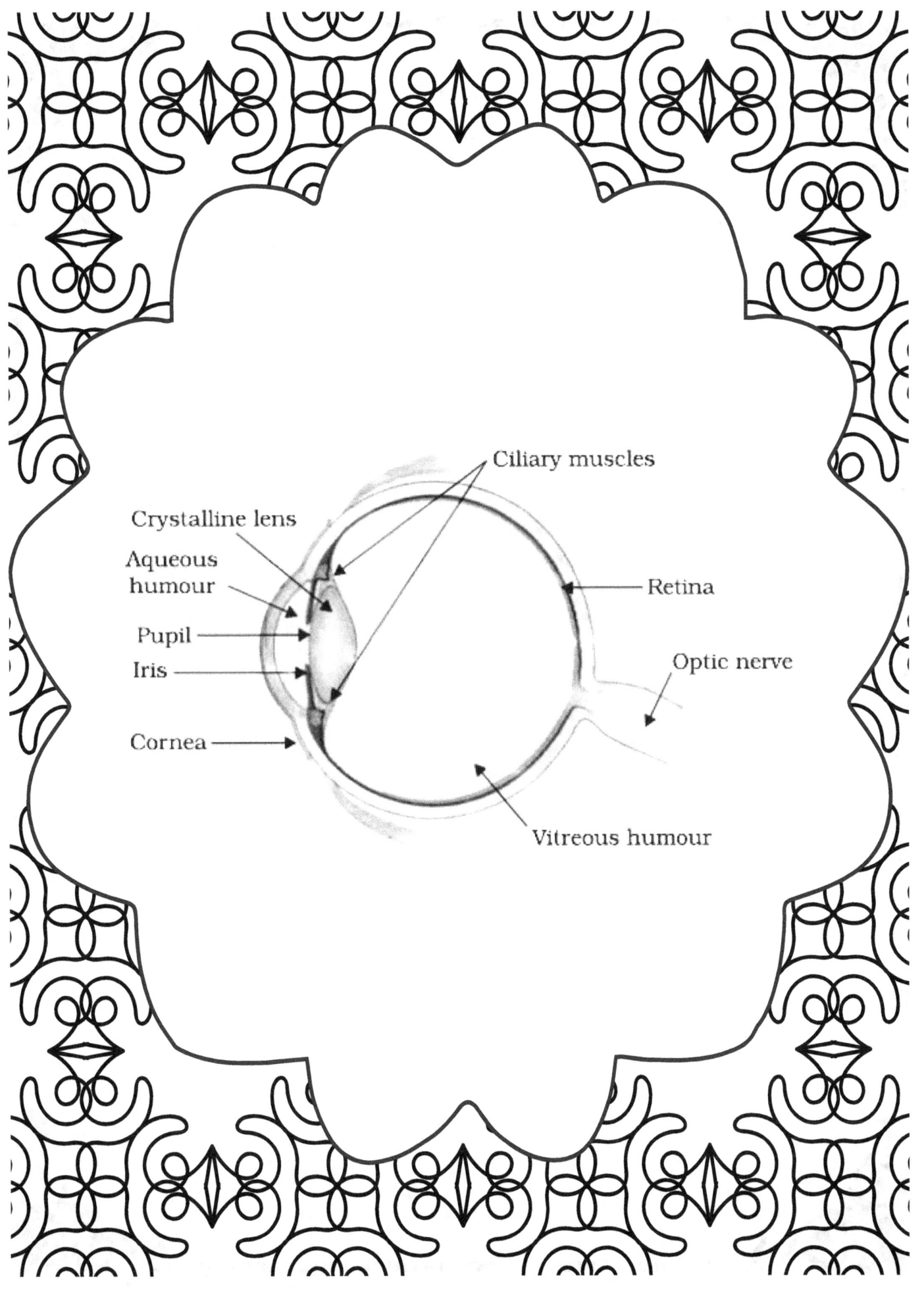

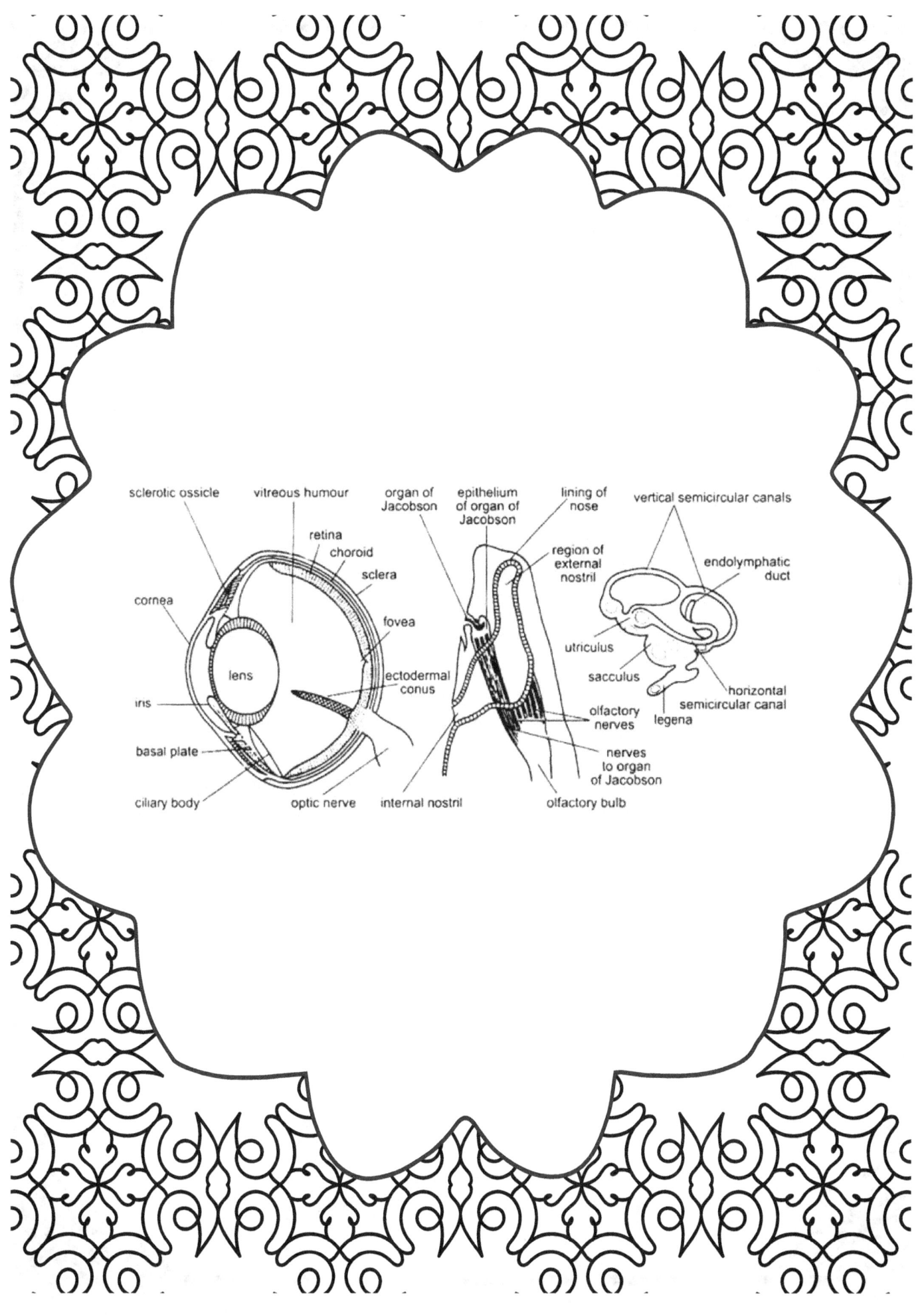

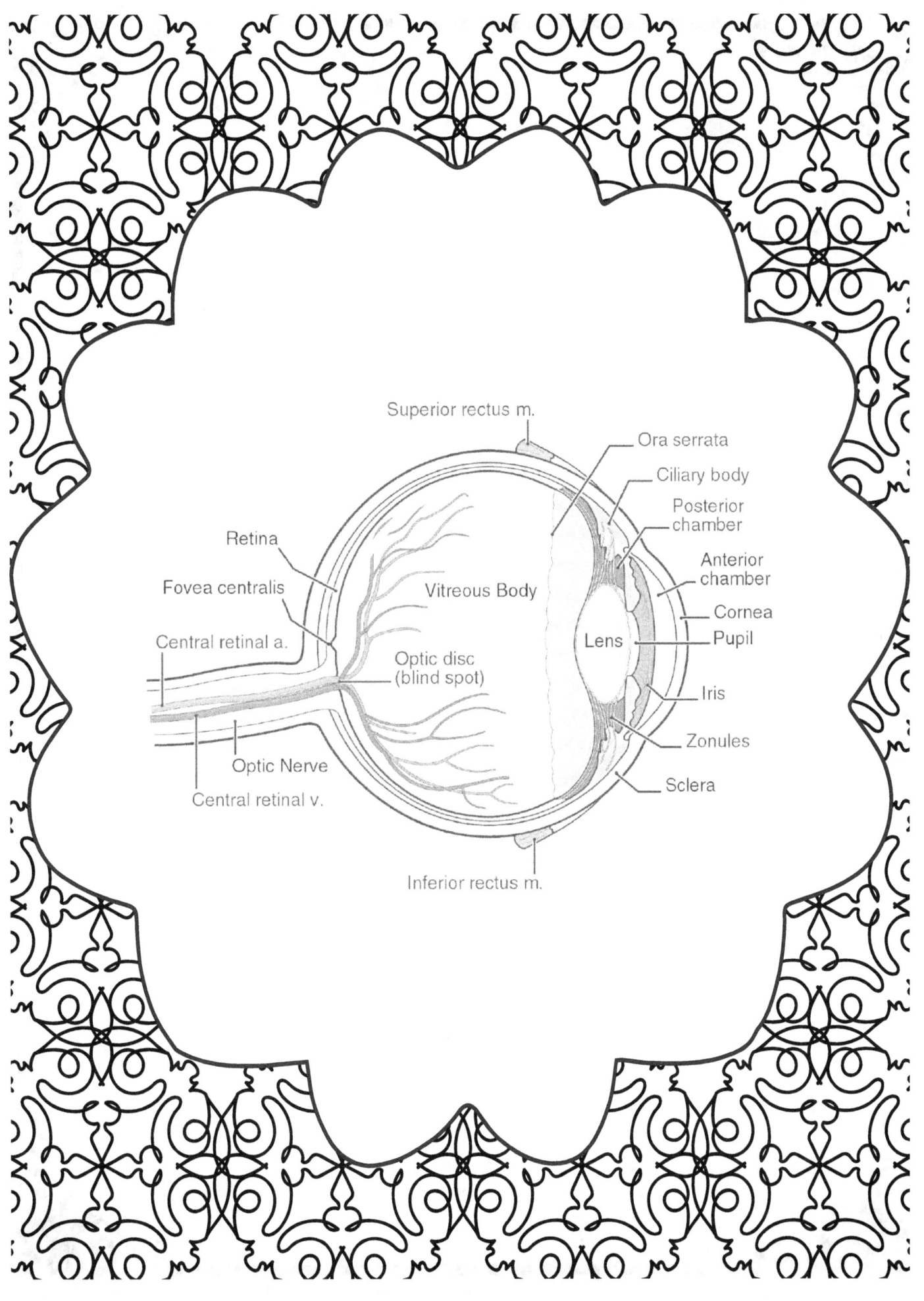

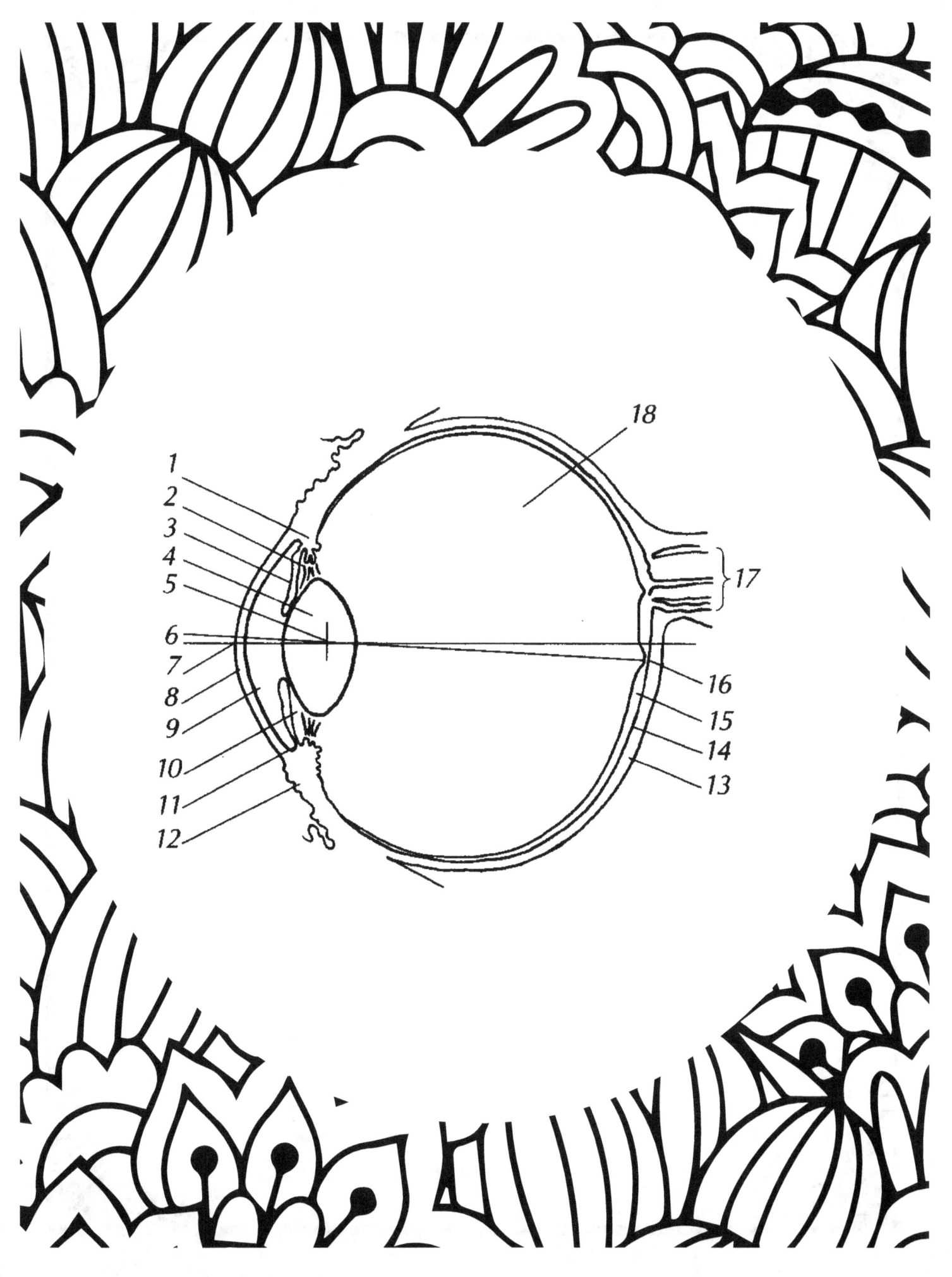

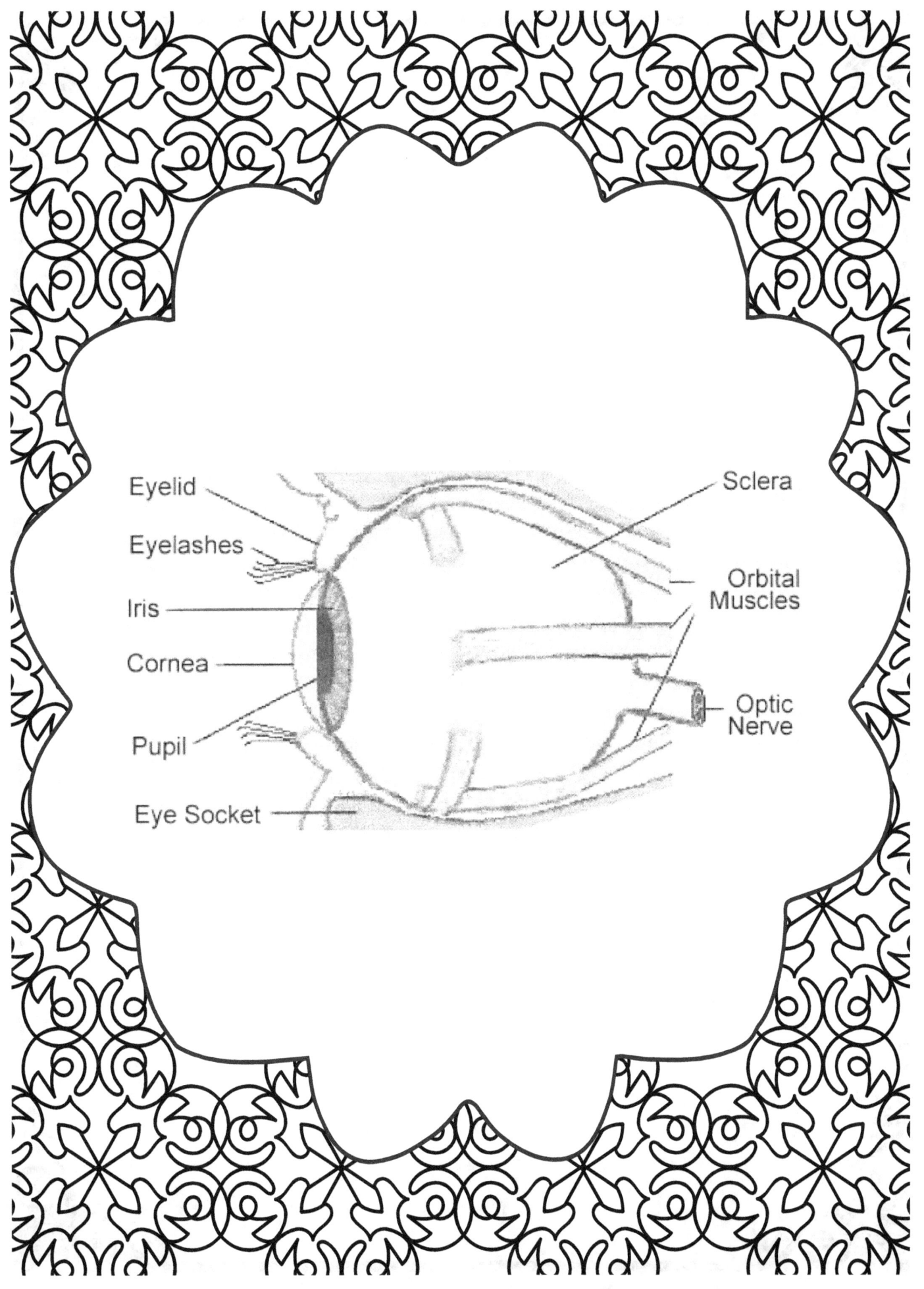

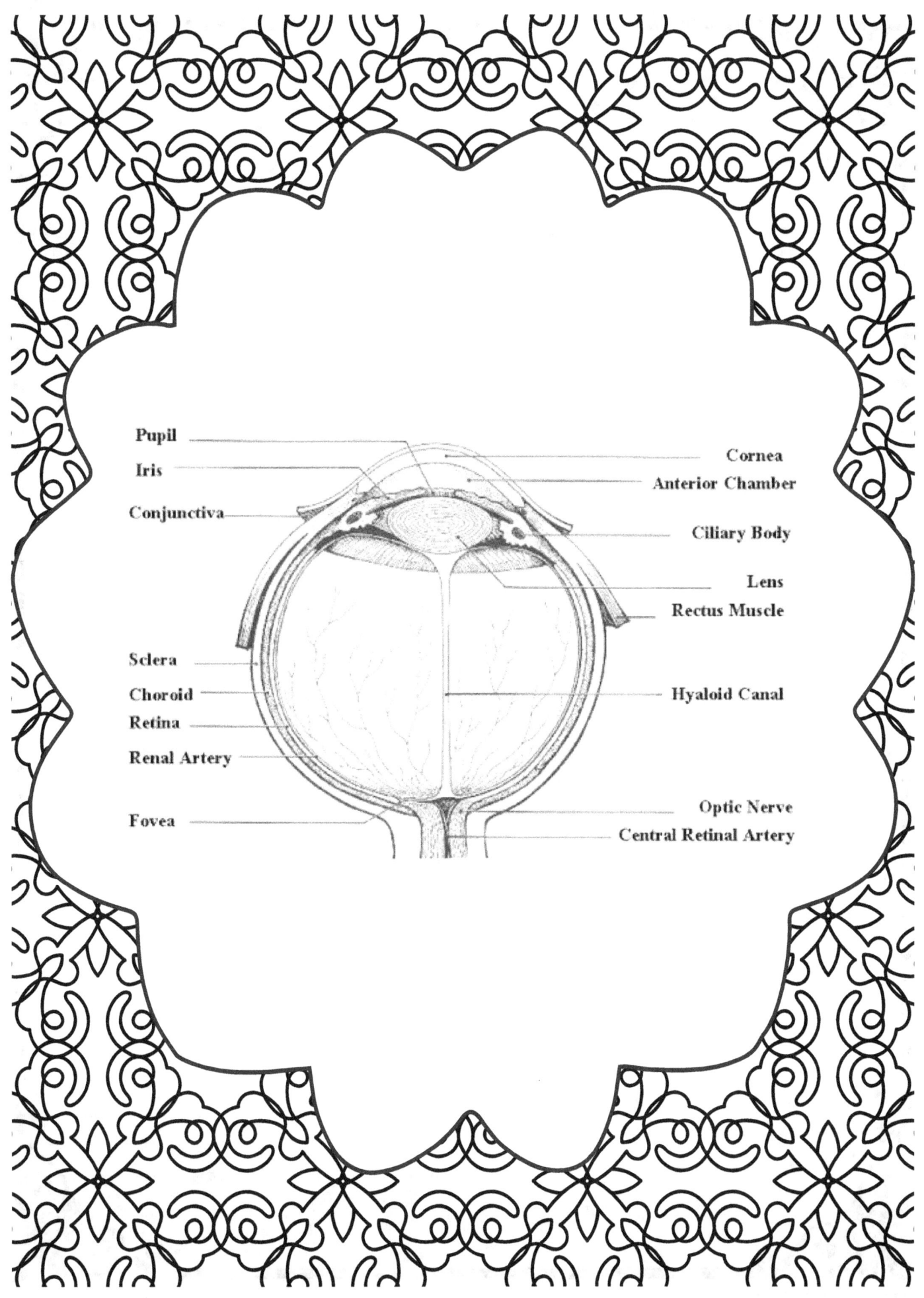

Pupil

Iris

Conjunctiva

Sclera

Choroid

Retina

Renal Artery

Fovea

Cornea

Anterior Chamber

Ciliary Body

Lens

Rectus Muscle

Hyaloid Canal

Optic Nerve

Central Retinal Artery

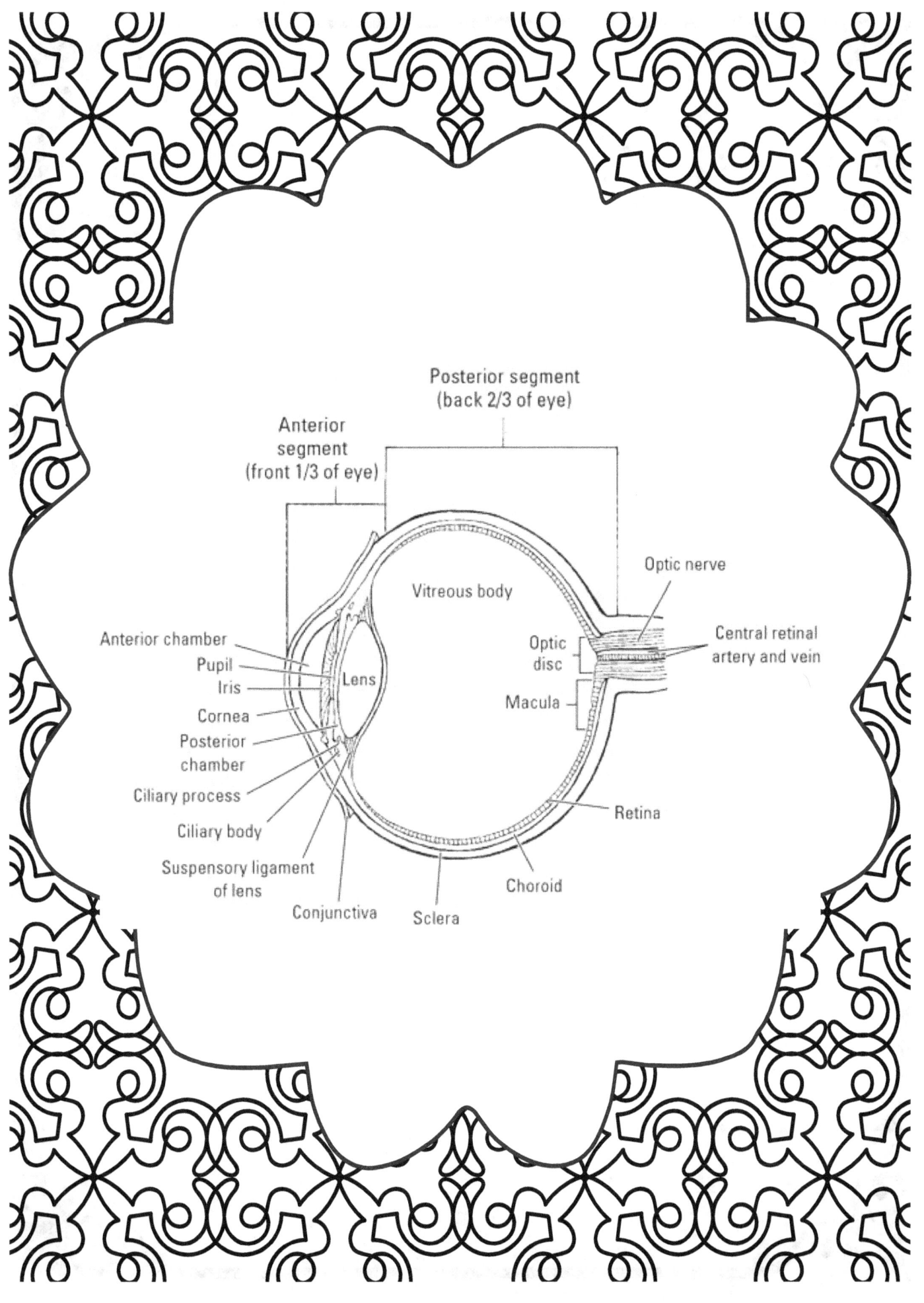

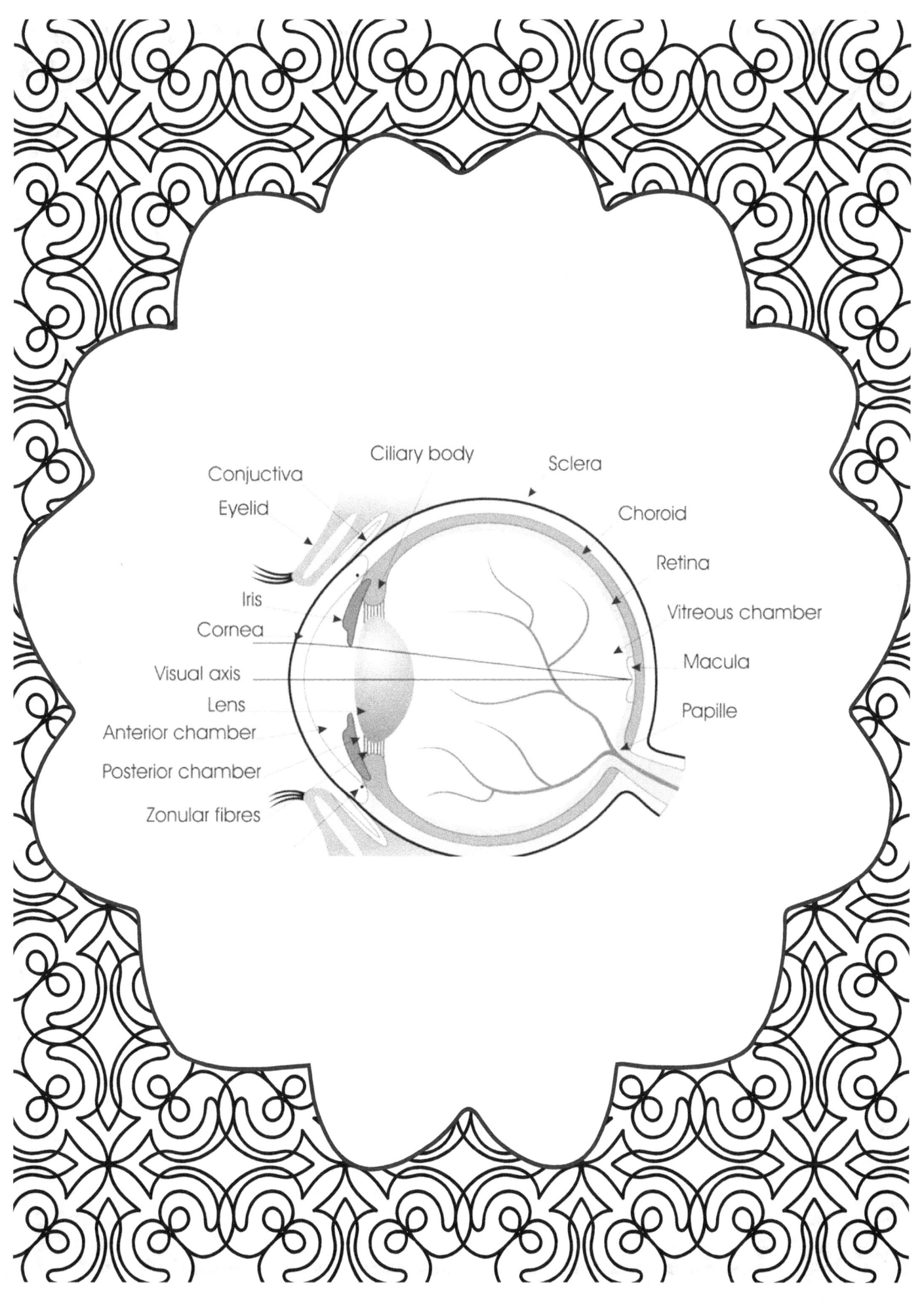

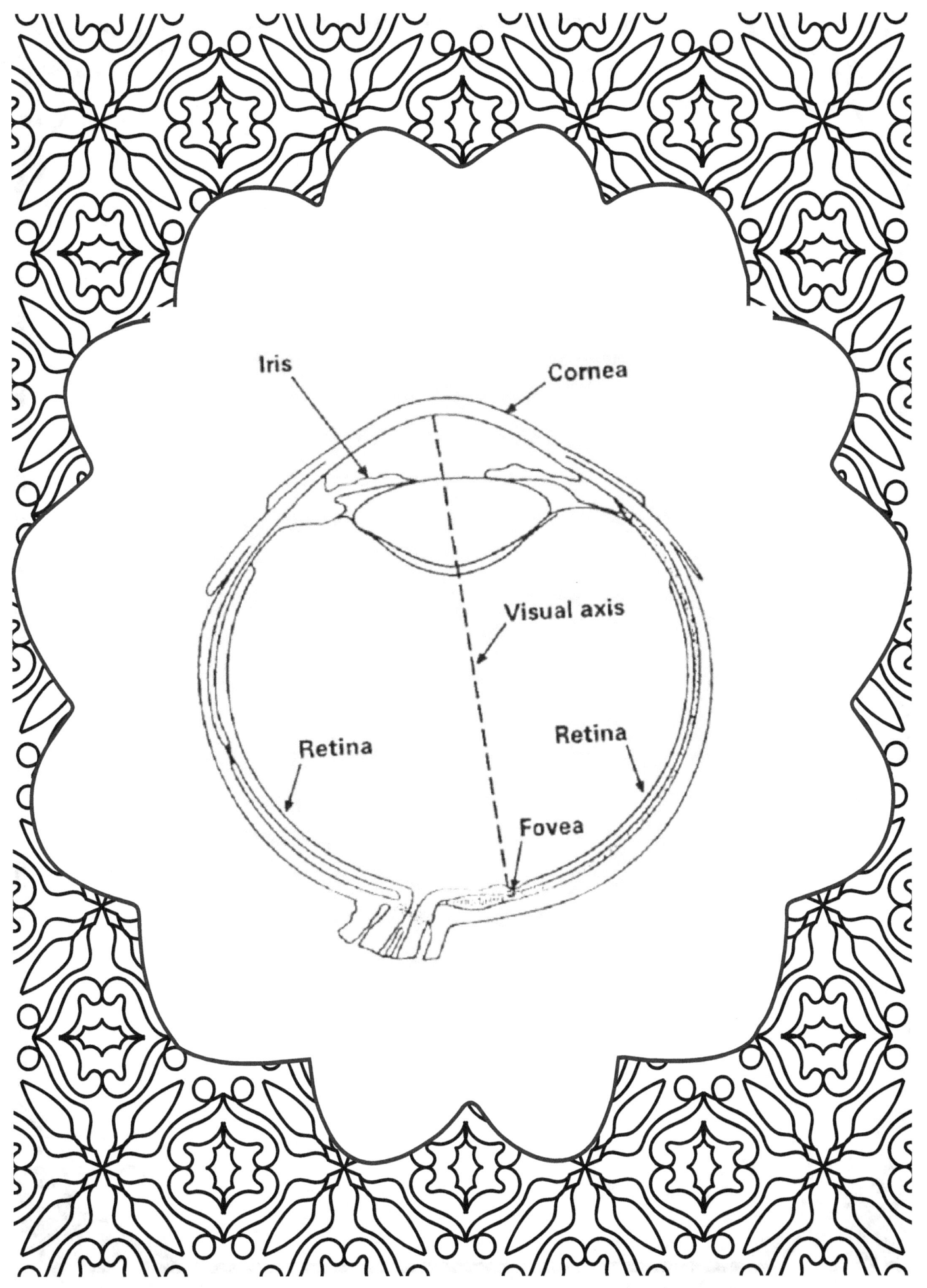

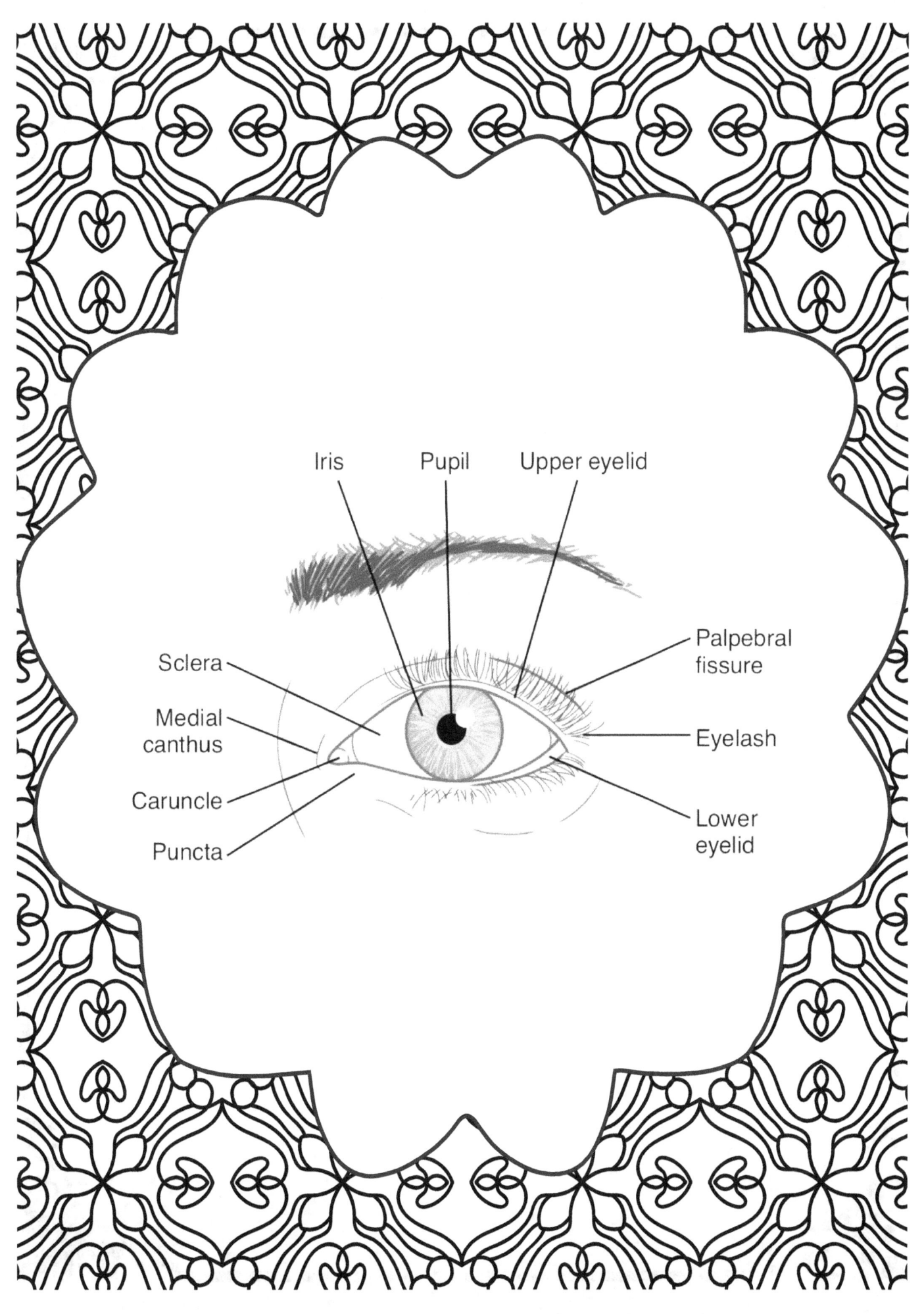

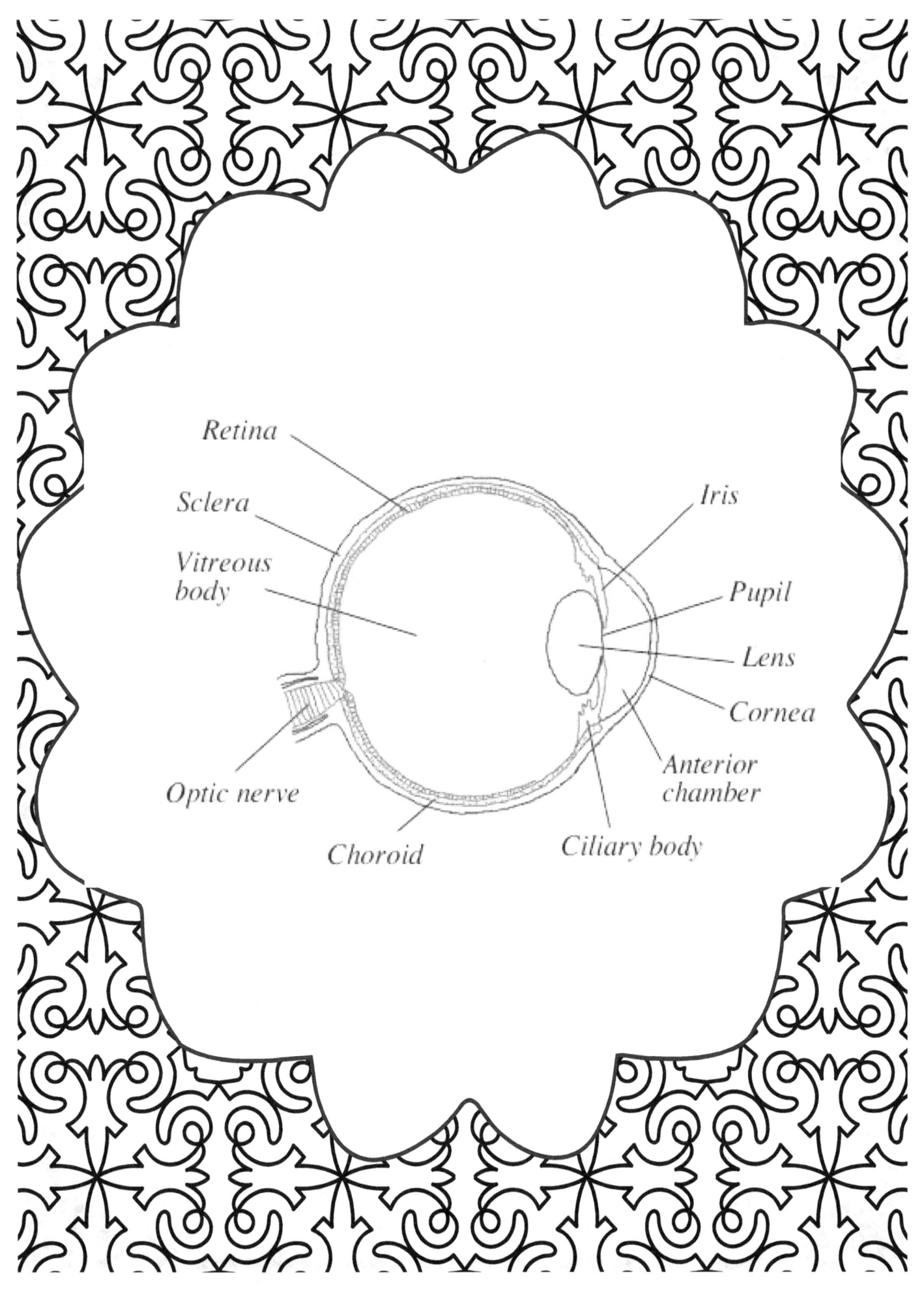

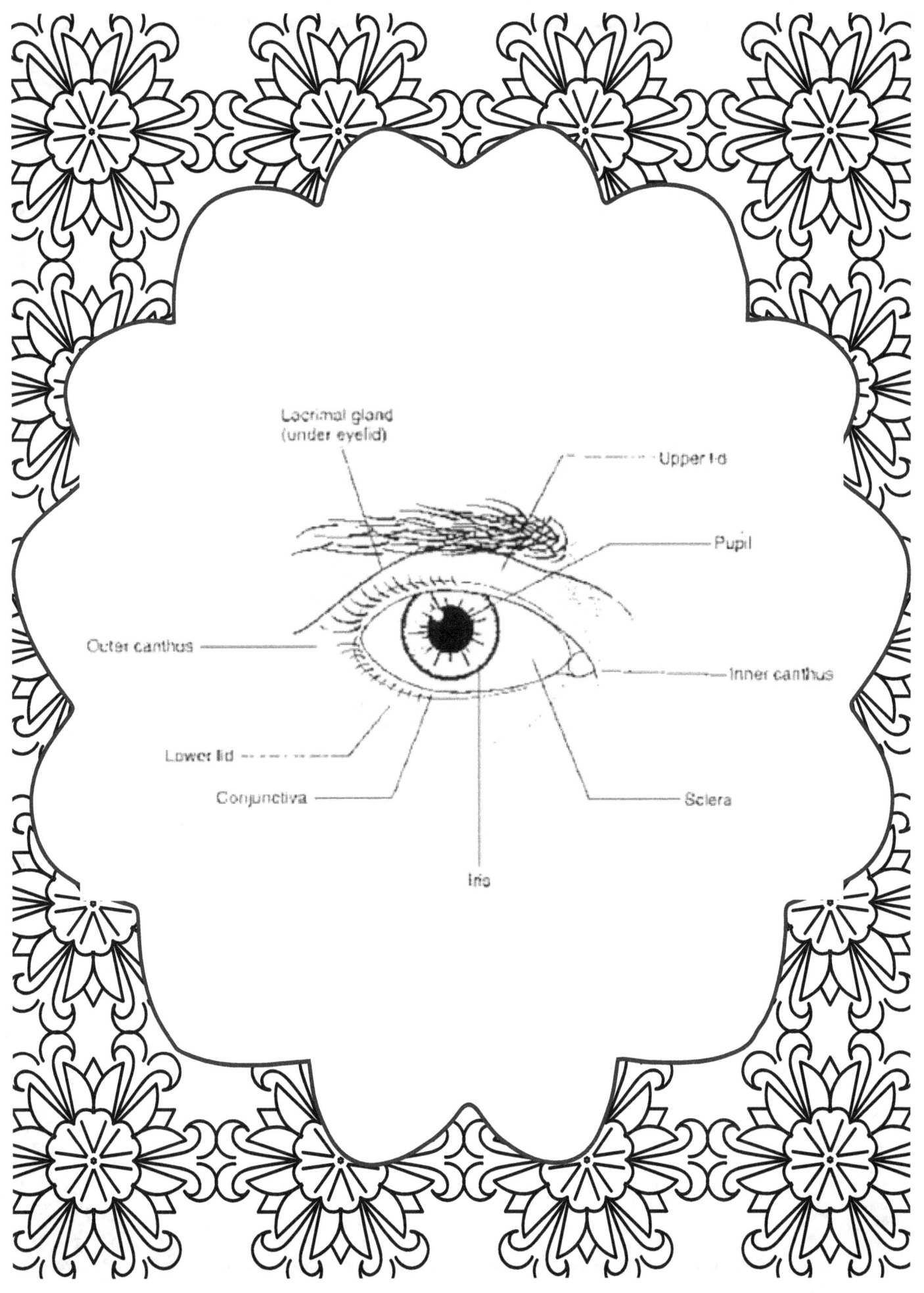

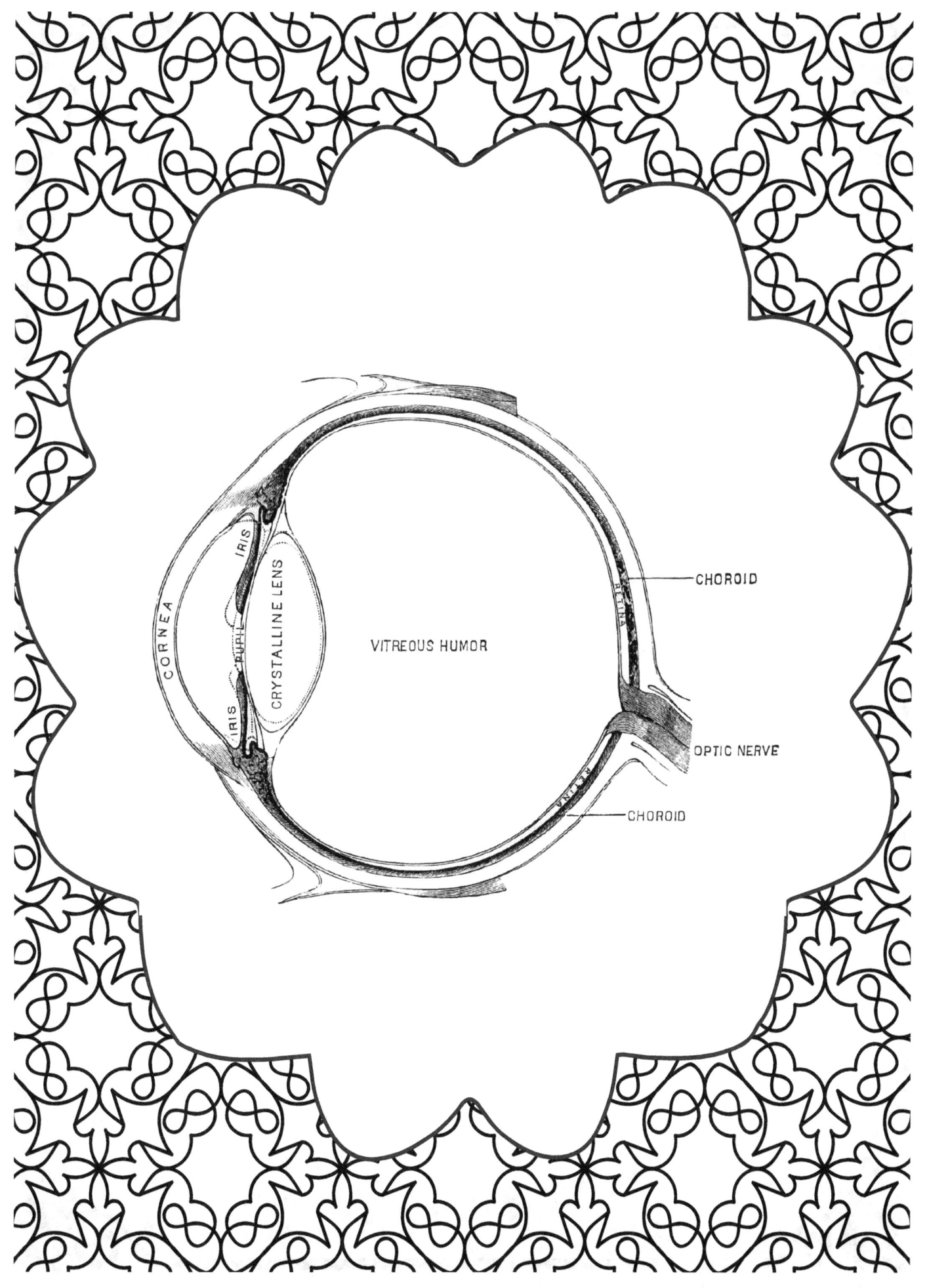

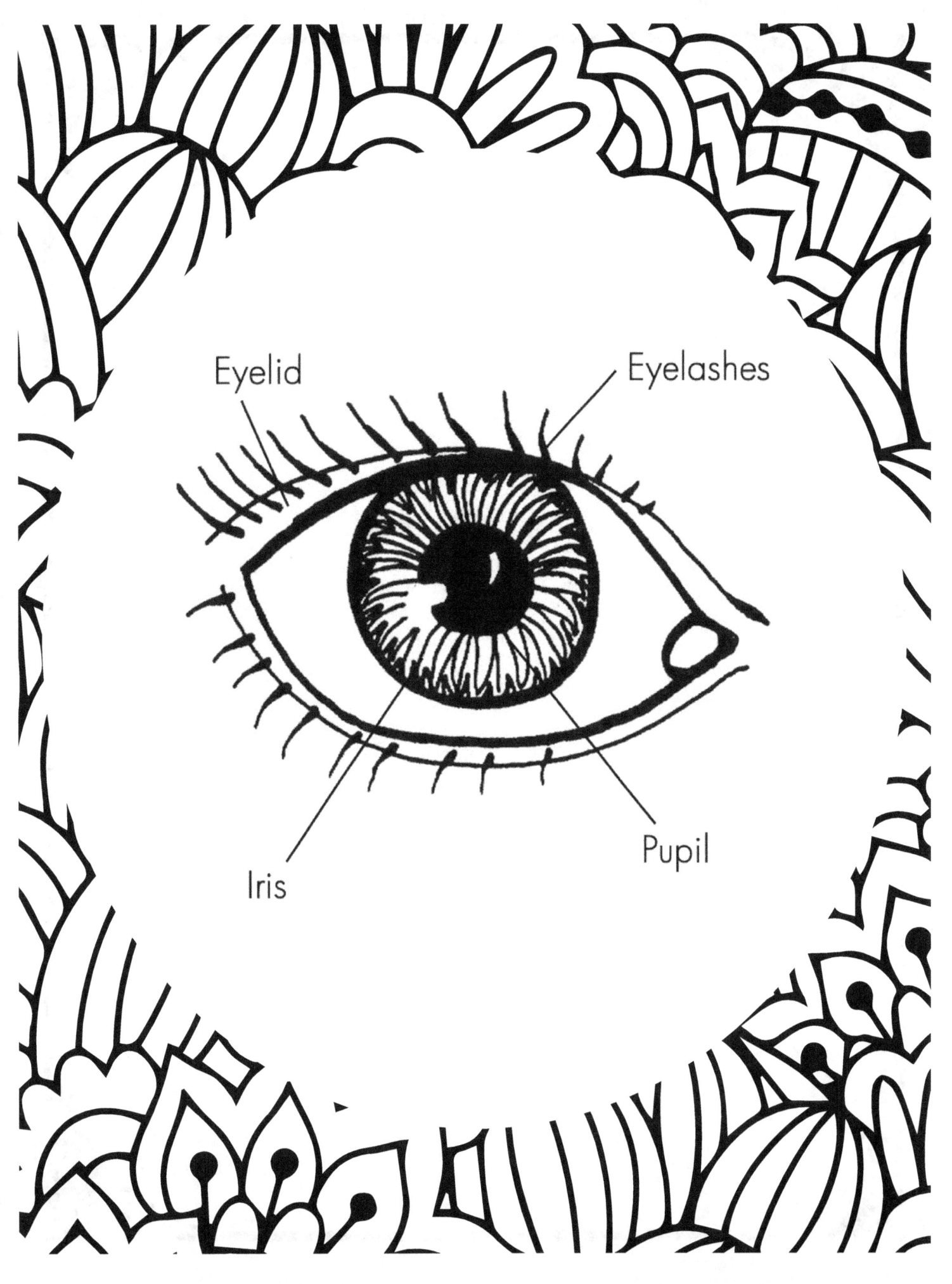

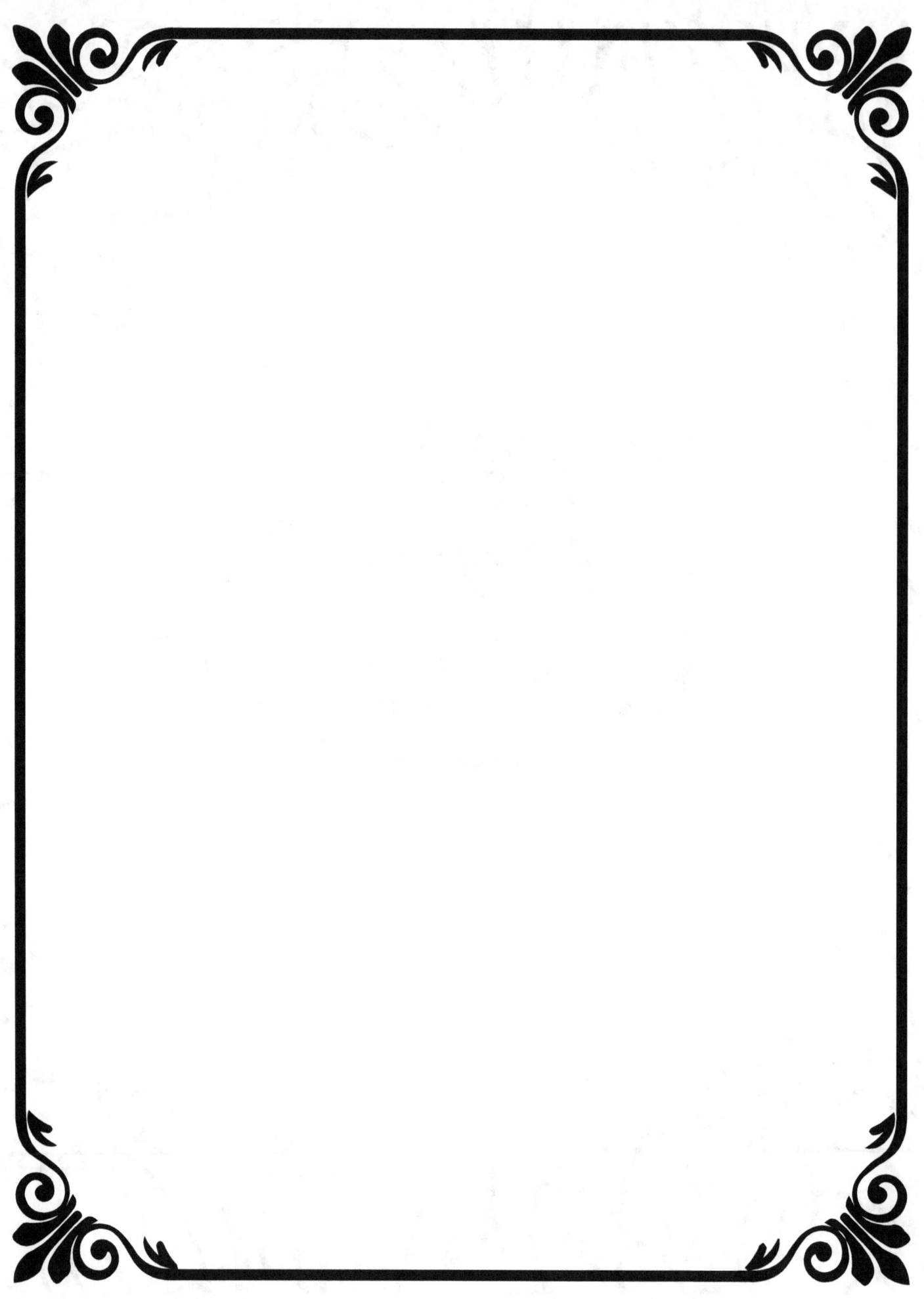

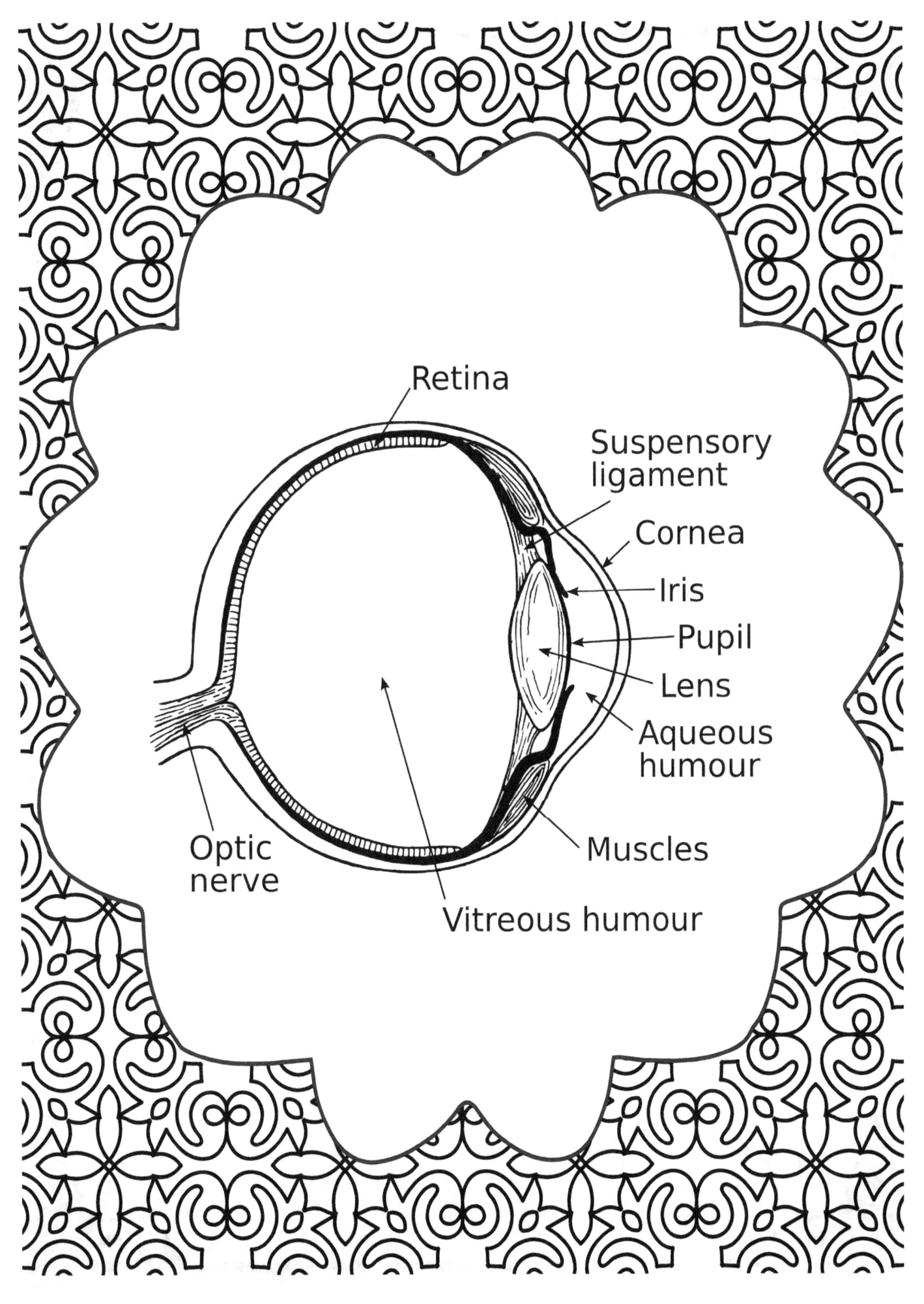

Retina

Suspensory
ligament

Cornea

Iris

Pupil

Lens

Aqueous
humour

Muscles

Optic
nerve

Vitreous humour

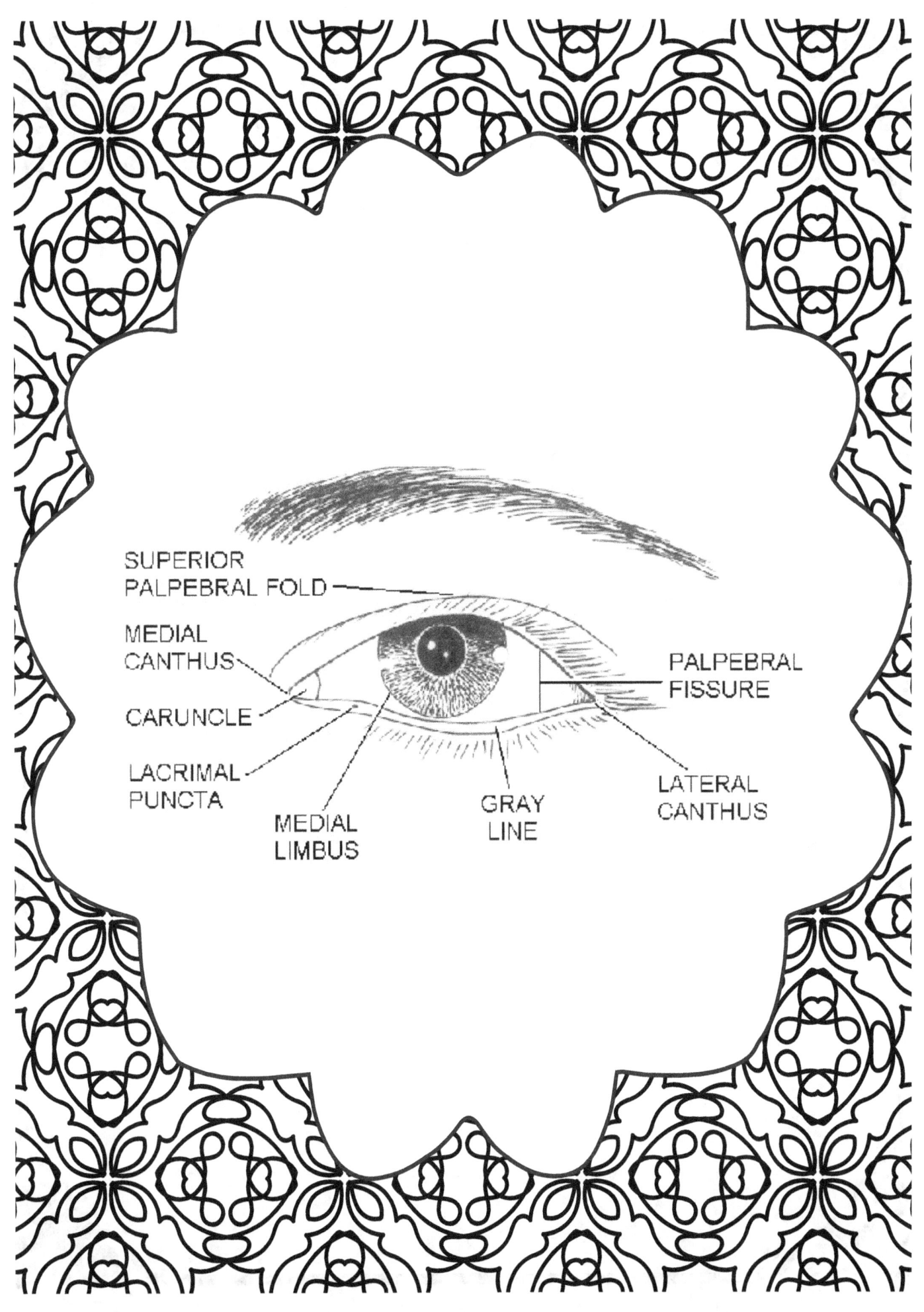

SUPERIOR
PALPEBRAL FOLD

MEDIAL
CANTHUS

CARUNCLE

LACRIMAL
PUNCTA

MEDIAL
LIMBUS

GRAY
LINE

PALPEBRAL
FISSURE

LATERAL
CANTHUS

EYE ANATOMY

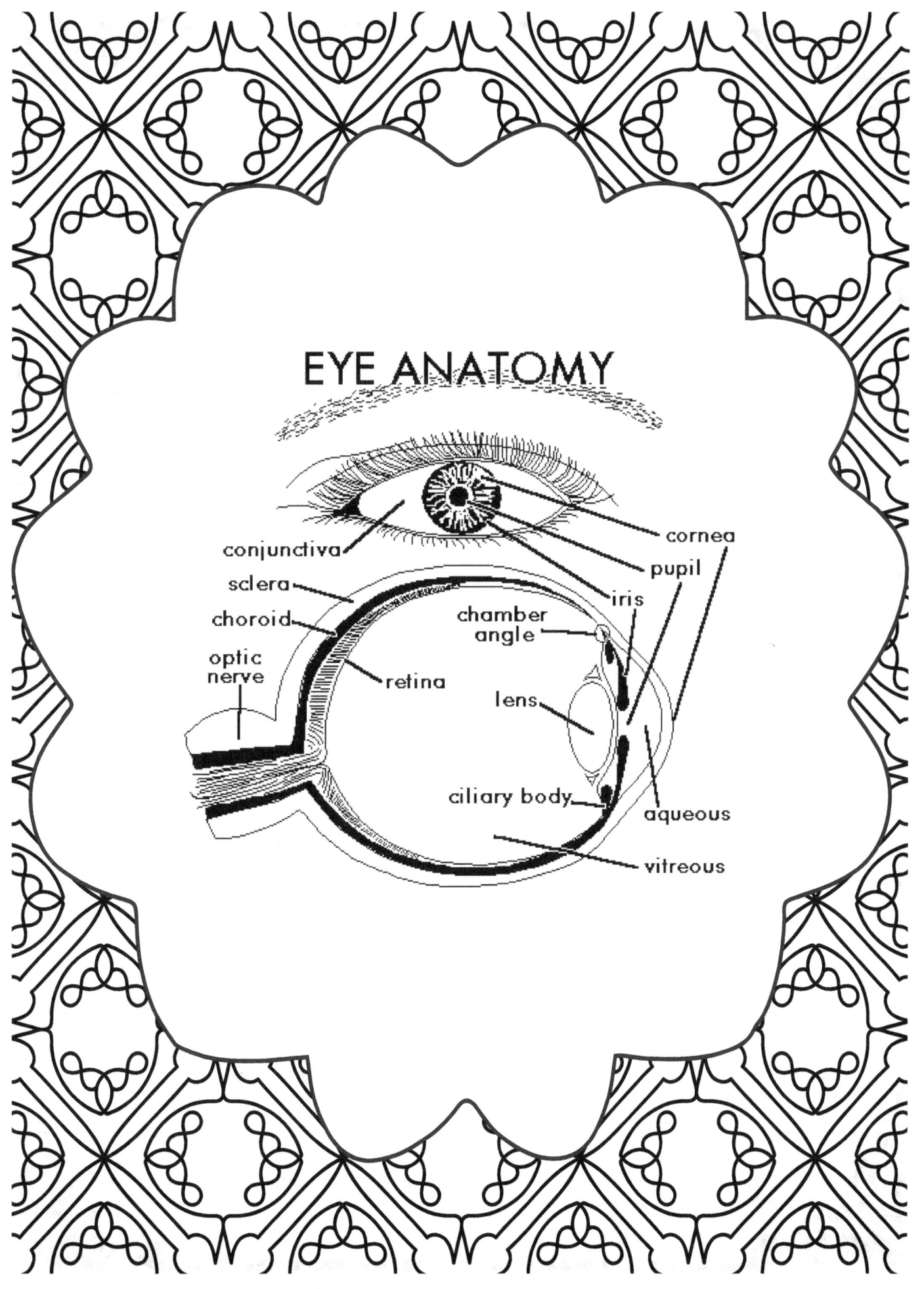

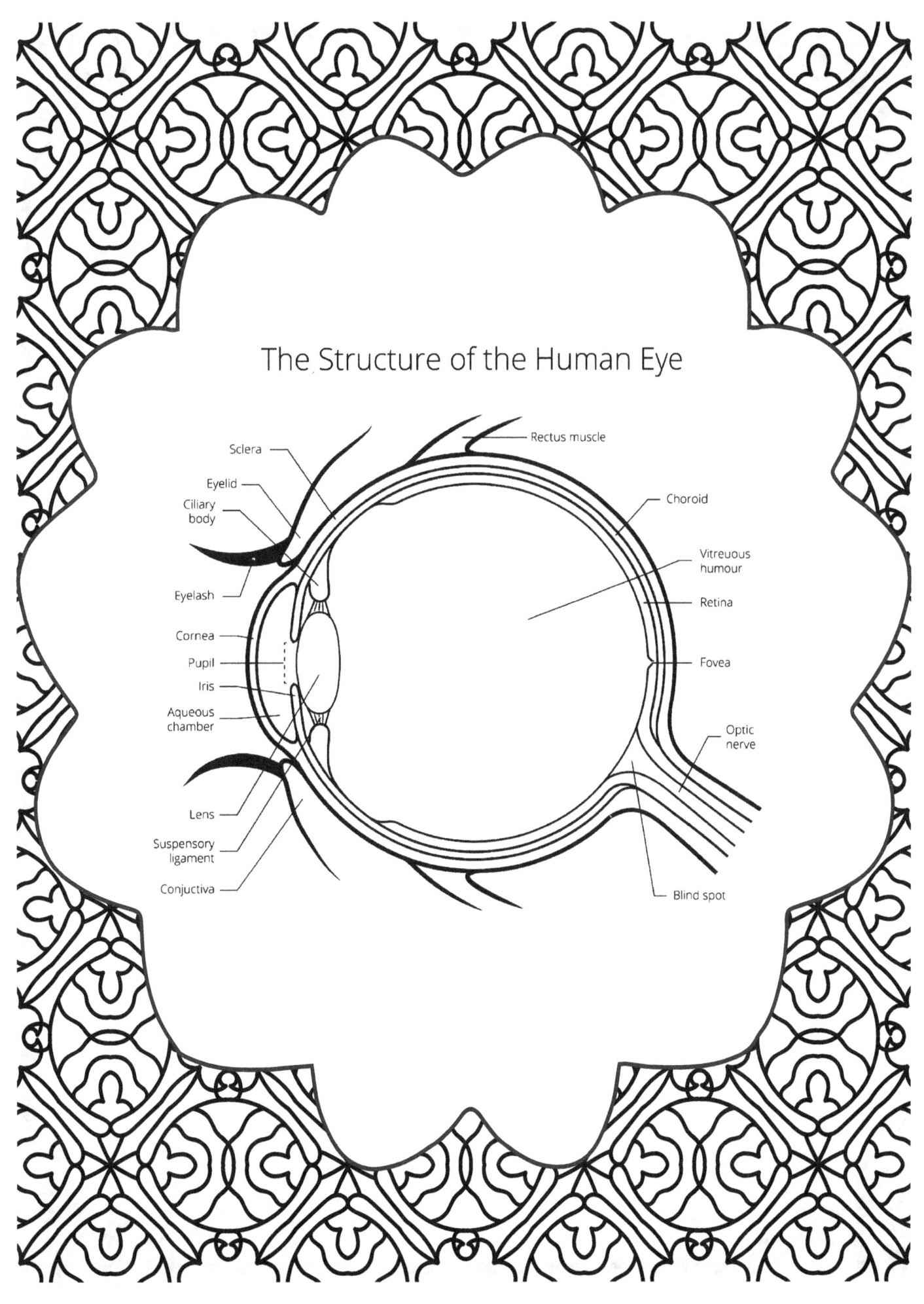

The Structure of the Human Eye

Sclera

Eyelid

Ciliary body

Eyelash

Cornea

Pupil

Iris

Aqueous chamber

Lens

Suspensory ligament

Conjuctiva

Rectus muscle

Choroid

Vitreuous humour

Retina

Fovea

Optic nerve

Blind spot

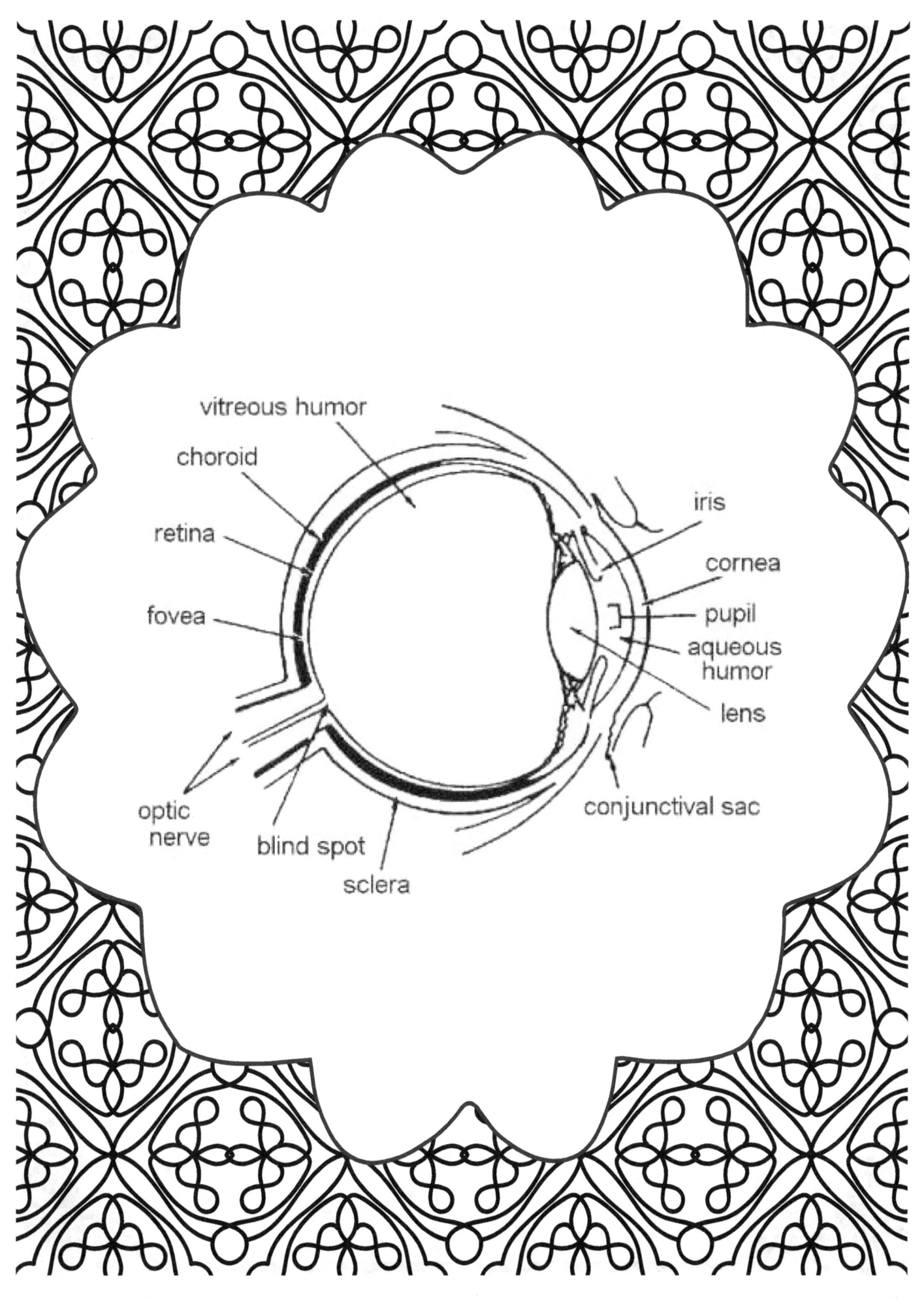

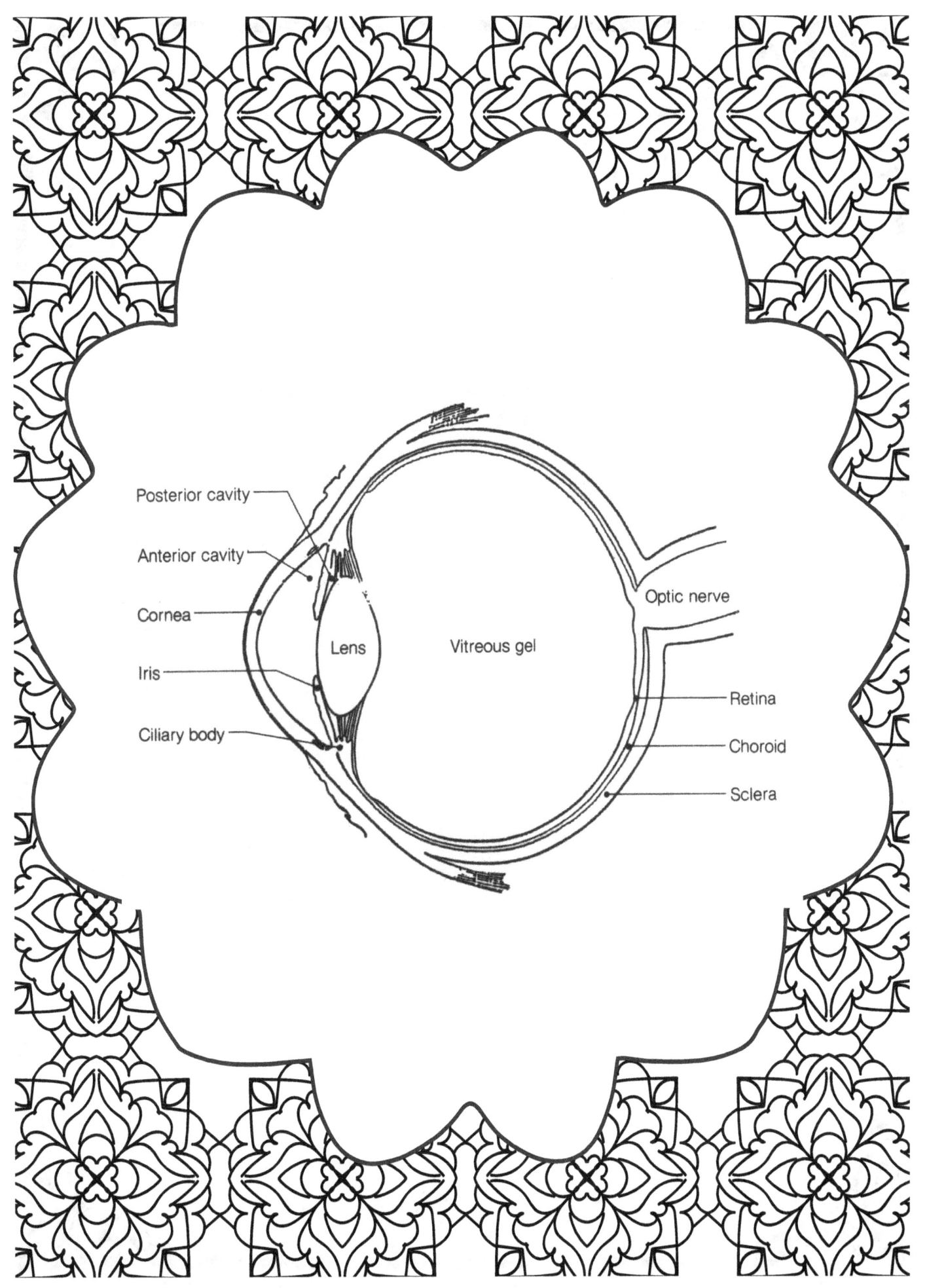

Posterior cavity

Anterior cavity

Cornea

Iris

Ciliary body

Lens

Vitreous gel

Optic nerve

Retina

Choroid

Sclera

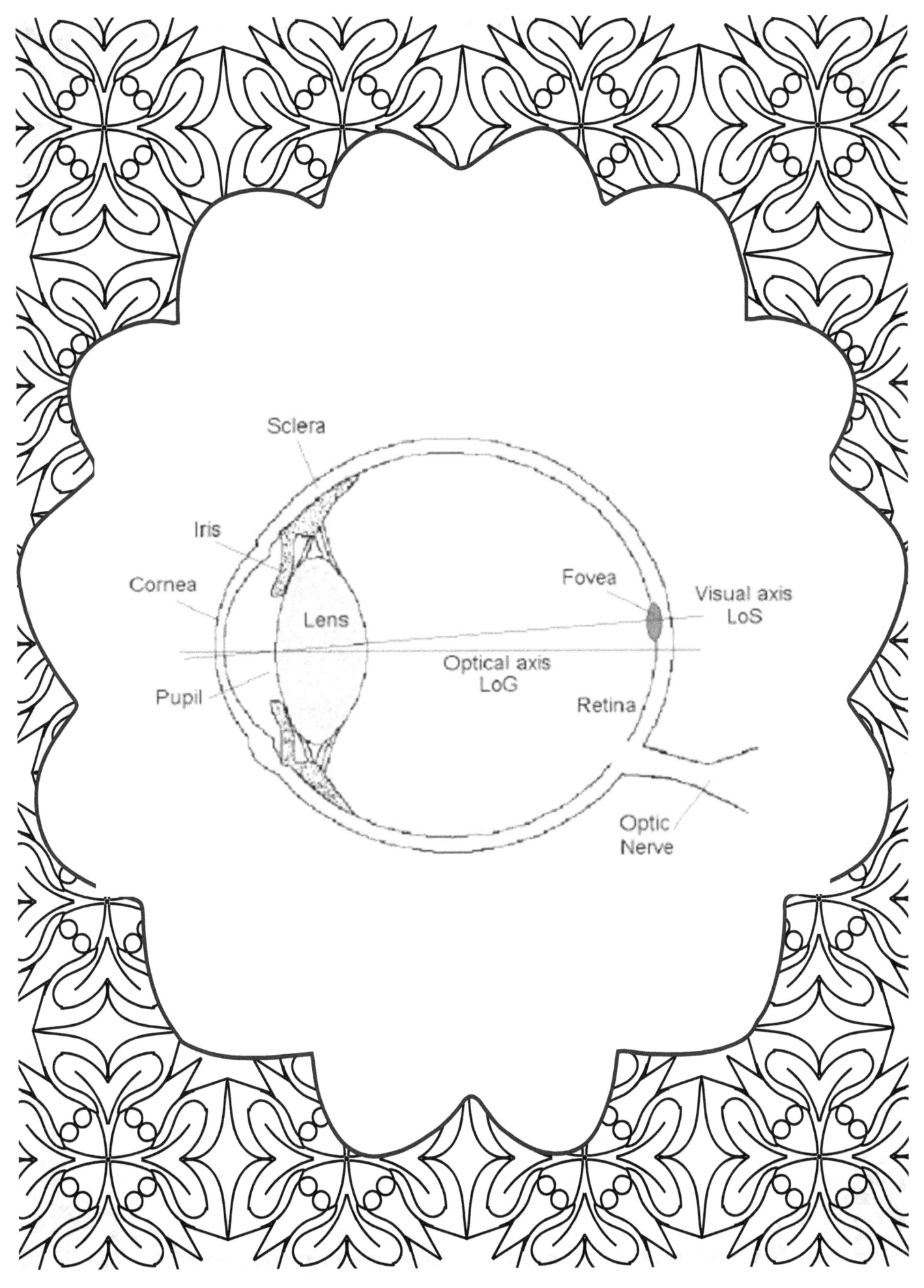

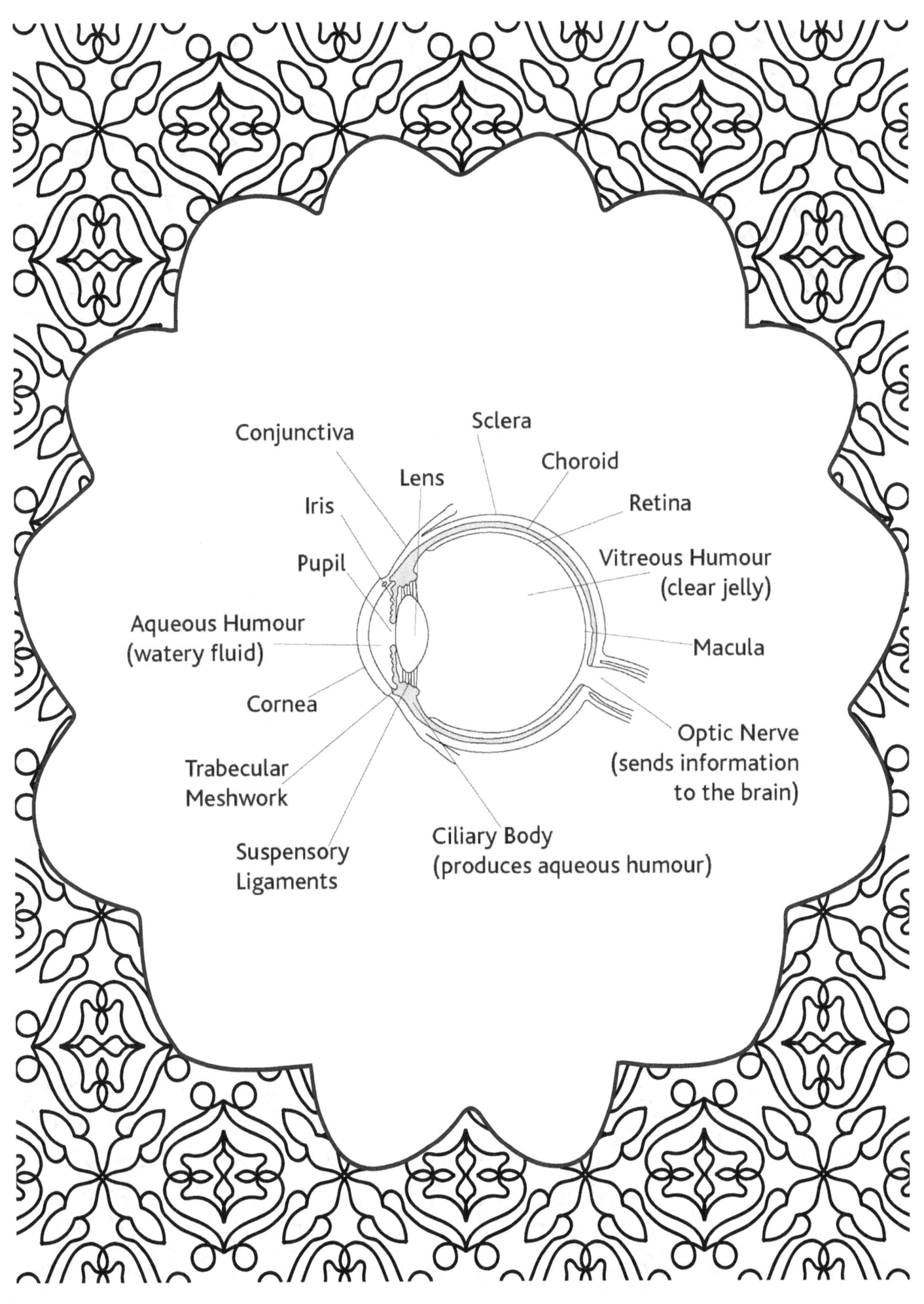

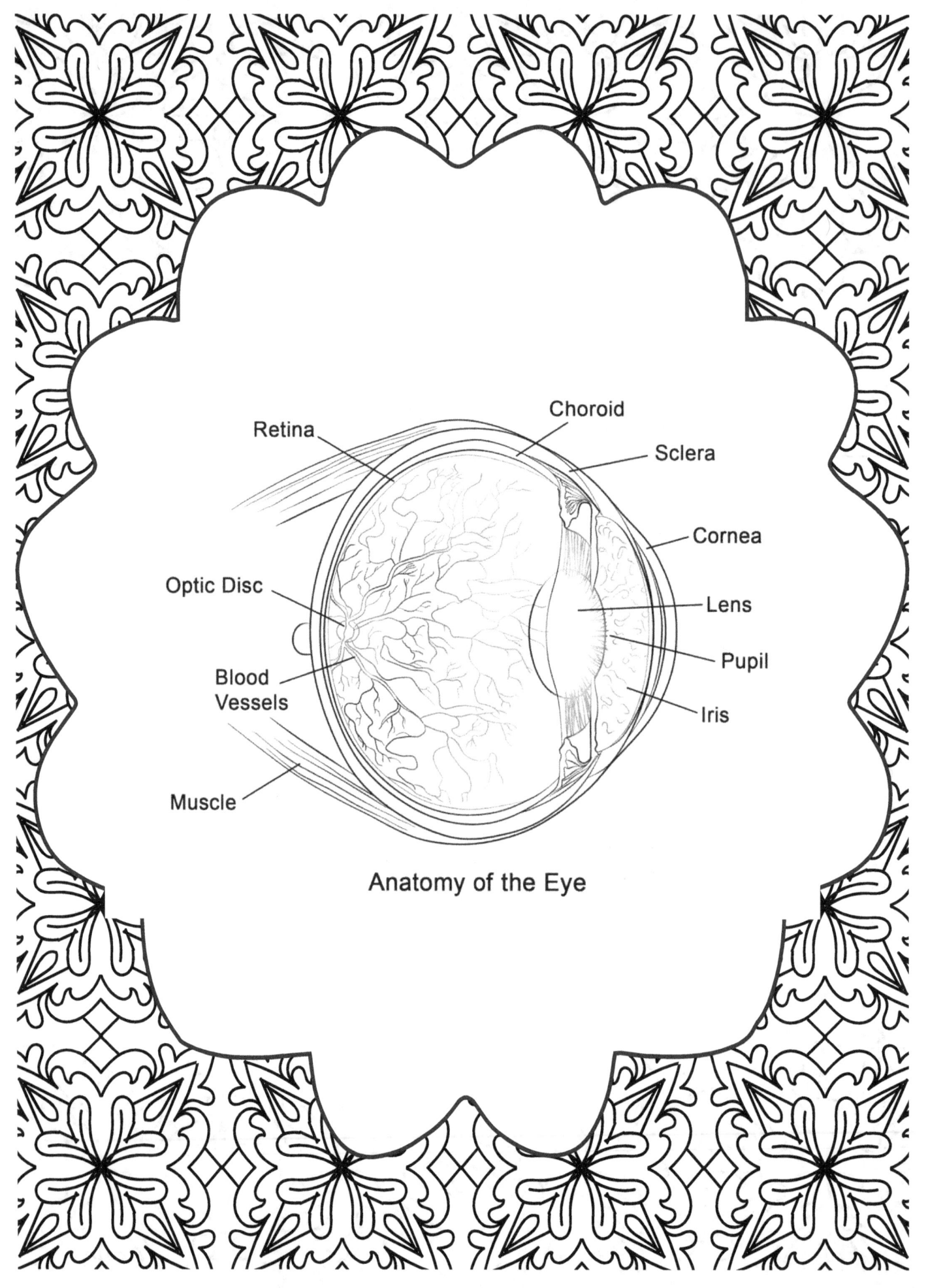

Anatomy of the Eye